Interfacing Immunity, Gut Health and Performance

Interfacing Immunity, Gut Health and Performance

Edited by

LA Tucker and JA Taylor-Pickard

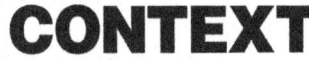

Context Products Ltd
53 Mill Street, Packington
Leicestershire, LE65 1WN, United Kingdom

First published 2004
Reprinted 2013
© The several contributors names in the list of contents

British Library Cataloguing in Publication Data
Interfacing Immunity, Gut Health and Performance
I. Tucker, L.A., II. Taylor-Pickard, J.A.

ISBN 978-1-899043-53-8

Disclaimer

Every reasonable effort has been made to ensure that the material in this book is true, correct, complete and appropriate at the time of writing. Nevertheless, the publishers and authors do not accept responsibility for any omission or error, or for any injury, damage, loss or financial consequences arising from the use of the book.

Typeset by Context Products Ltd

CONTENTS

Introduction

In the last decade, commercial animal nutritionists have found it increasingly difficult to keep up to date with developments in sciences relating to their field. Many who visit conferences regularly find new topics of interest that would be rewarding and stimulating to explore. However the deluge of reading material in the form of magazines and journals, not to mention the larger corporate workload generated by advances in communications, make it even harder to justify spending scant reading time on 'peripheral' subjects.

It is recognised that the cross- pollination of ideas from related subject areas have a major impact on successful development and commercialisation of feed and nutrition products and improved practice within animal production systems. In order to attain exposure to a diversity of sciences, useful summaries related in plain language are essential. The opportunity to devote a single day at a dedicated seminar covering such topics is a highly useful and efficient way of learning more about these subjects.

To this end, the following collection of papers were gathered together and presented at a seminar held for pig and poultry nutritionists in 2004. The aim of this exercise was to give delegates an overview of important topics relevant to animal production, including the fast moving and complex science of immunology, that (especially for those without specialist molecular biology training) can be difficult to follow.

The fields of nutrition, animal physiology, gut development, microbial gut flora and immunology are intrinsically linked, as they are directly influenced by each other. The 'combined' approach in terms of understanding the relationship between different factors and the overall impact on animal health, welfare and production is replacing the old approach where one cause has one effect. We now know that many diseases and production problems are multi-factorial and are dependant upon other predisposing influences. It is therefore essential that the modern animal producer and feed nutritionist has a basic, current understanding of related sciences, in order to best apply new methods of improving animal performance and welfare.

The following papers build up a comprehensive understanding of these interactions, from production considerations and the analysis of potential future problems, through the current research into gut development, microbial populations and immunity, and how these interact with feed and feed ingredients. As a seminar series, these topics generated great interest amongst the many delegates from a spectrum of monogastric commercial operations from different parts of the world. I trust that readers of the papers will also find them as stimulating.

Dr Lucy Tucker
Dr Julie Taylor-Pickard
May 2004

Future challenges in poultry meat production

Steve Leeson
Department of Animal and Poultry Science, University of Guelph, Guelph, Ontario N1G 2W1, Canada

Introduction

The poultry meat industry has undergone remarkable change and growth over the last 30 yrs, and it seems that this will continue in the next 10-20 years. The meat industry has undoubtedly been the most successful, yet the egg industry is now making strides in new product development. Today, we see 4 kg male broilers at 49 d of age. There is often debate about there being an end point to this increased genetic potential, yet the geneticists indicate that selection pressure will be little reduced in the foreseeable future.

The modern broiler chicken continues to show increased yearly genetic gains, that equates to almost 1 d reduction in time taken for males to achieve 2.5 kg live weight. This increased growth potential (Figure 1) has meant that we are continually increasing our global consumption of broiler meat, since bird numbers are also increasing annually.

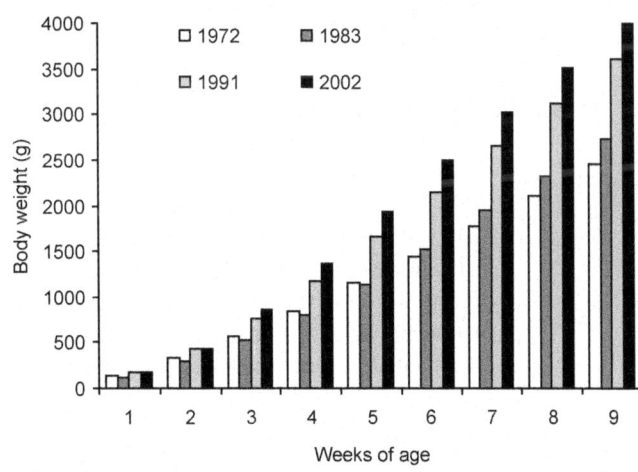

Figure 1. Male broiler growth over the past 30 years.

World production

In 2015 there is a prediction for consumption of around 65million tons of broiler meat, which equates to a yearly live production of 85 million tons or about 43 billion 2 kg birds. The industry will require some 155 million tons of feed at a value of close to $33 billion. These statistics assume a more moderate annual growth of about 1 million tons live bird annual increase.

There will likely be a change in location of this future production. Currently we have major production centres in the Americas, Europe and Asia. The Americas and Asia will continue to meet world demand, while Europe seems destined to supply its own local market for niche products. Within the Americas, the USA and Brazil will continue to be the major producers and exporters while in Asia China will be the most important area of production. It is obvious that while it is possible to produce broilers in almost any geographical region, it is the location of ever more sophisticated processing facilities that dictate major centres of production. Some countries will continue with marketing of live birds (e.g. Mexico and Peru) and while this effectively excludes imports, it does limit future expansion and profitability. Processing and further processing are the keys to market penetration of poultry meat, and these facilities are becoming increasingly expensive to establish and maintain. The current trend to producing heavier birds is merely a response to reducing processing costs per unit of meat yield. However there are current limits to how heavy we can economically grow birds. The limiting factor to processing in the next 20 years will be an adequate and economical supply of water that meets ever-increasing standards for pollutants and contaminants. We will meet these standards by utilizing water purification systems, which will necessarily add to our cost of production.

Bird type and genetics

There will be no major change in emphasis for genetic selection in the near future. Over the past 20 years we have seen a 25-50 g increase in weight of 42-49d old broilers and this trend will continue in the foreseeable future. There is an obvious limit to this growth potential that is fuelled by the bird's appetite, and the most likely reason being problems with skeletal and cardio-vascular systems. There are also concerns about the effectiveness of immature digestive systems.

The heritability for growth characteristics is quite high, being in the order of 0.4 - 0.6. This means that progress can be made by simply selecting the heaviest birds in a flock as breeders. For this trend to be maintained over future generations, the primary breeders have to continually find individuals within their pedigree lines, that are 100-200 g heavier than average. Anyone who handles and weighs individual birds knows that such individuals exist; yet finding enough 'fit' individuals each generation becomes increasingly difficult. Currently in small experimental male flocks, averaging 2.7 kg at 42d, we see individuals weighing 3.2 or even 3.5 kg, and so variation still exists. In fact, at our research facilities we are becoming more concerned with bird-to-bird variation, which seems to be increasing, and is making the identification of various treatment effects more difficult. This variation is present at 7d of age, and is becoming more obvious over time.

Meat yield, and especially that of breast meat, has become a major factor in selection of male line breeder candidates. The emphasis on breast yield has been fuelled by the premium realized for this meat in North America, a situation that often does not occur in other countries. Interestingly, today in North America the premium for white meat over dark meat is less than it was just 5 years ago, although companies still find it challenging to realize economic returns on dark meat.

In considering genetic programs for broilers, one cannot ignore the need for efficient breeder characteristics. Carte (1986) eloquently detailed this comparison for broiler versus breeder traits within a genetic selection program (Table 1). These data have been modified to reflect economics more current in 2004.

Table 1.
Relative economic values within an integrated broiler operation, where costs are equivalent to about 1¢/kg live weight.

Bird Type	Performance
A. Broiler traits:	+0.19 kg live weight -0.06 feed:gain +1.1% breast yield -1.2% condemnation -2.2% liveability
B. Broiler breeder traits:	+32 hatching eggs +17% hatchability all eggs set -1.6 kg feed/dozen eggs -15¢/dozen hatching eggs -17 kg breeder feed

Adapted from Carte (1986)

These data suggest that, all other factors remaining the same, then a +0.19 kg increase in live weight at a specific market age will reduce overall costs by 1¢/kg broiler live weight produced. Increasing breast yield by 1.1% has the same economic benefit etc. Of particular interest are the relatively large changes that have to occur at the breeder level in order to bring about the same economic return. Over the next 10 years or so, the industry cannot expect any major change in breeder performance.

Broiler production systems

There has been substantial consolidation in the type of housing and construction systems of broiler facilities used worldwide. Anyone building new facilities today will likely design individual sites for at least 100,000 birds. These houses will be fully controlled environment or "open-sided" with more elaborate insulated curtains, incorporating tunnel ventilation. With additional help during catching and clean out, mechanized systems allow for one person to manage at least 100,000 birds, and so this becomes the approximate minimal economic size for newer construction. We will not likely see any further reduction in labour input, assuming that we wish to practice good husbandry and have our birds inspected on a regular basis.

Another future challenge, is an adequate supply of 'clean' water for any broiler operation. In many regions, ground water levels are getting lower, which means more power required to pump to surface levels. In arable regions, the levels of minerals and pesticides will become more critical as a consequence of their gradual (20-30 year) movement through soil, and our inevitable advances in being able to detect ever-decreasing quantities residues (parts per trillion) of virtually any compound.

Feeding programs

Feed will always be the major input cost for broiler meat production. Corn and soybean meal will remain as a standard in broiler diets, and for this reason N. America and Brazil/Argentina will continue their dominance in production. There are really no major alternatives to corn and soybean meal on a worldwide basis. In certain regions, wheat is used because of artificial price support and/or artificial import tariffs on alternatives, and rice bran will continue to provide a niche role for diets in Asia. One often hears about 'new' alternate feed sources and by-products. Such discussion shows lack of understanding of world animal production, and whereas a few hundred tons of a 'new' by-product can be fitted into some local production system, there simply is not any undiscovered ingredient that is going to have an impact on the price of corn and soybean meal.

For the last 10 years at least, the world has had an abundance of cheap grains and vegetable proteins, and the broiler industry has capitalized on this situation. While corn and soybean meal will continue to be the main constituents of broiler feeds, the role of meat and poultry by-product meals and animal fats is less predictable. With Brazil/Argentina now being the major exporter of corn and soybeans, it is unlikely that we will see short supply of these ingredients in the near future. Even though there are only limited reserves of these ingredients, the seasonal supply from the USA and Brazil are likely to meet world demands.

The use of genetically modified cereals and vegetable proteins is another contentious issue. The general area of biotechnology and genetic engineering is still in its infancy, and will undoubtedly have a major impact on most aspects of agriculture and human medicine. It is unfortunate that the first commercial examples of this technology were seen to benefit only certain segments of society. Changing the nutrient profile of ingredients is not going to have a major effect on feeding broilers since if the bird's requirements do not change, then the net overall effect will be zero. For example, using a high lysine corn means that we will need less soybean meal or synthetic lysine. Modifying the nutrient level of plants will merely represent a net shift in the supply of individual nutrients, assuming these are cost effective substitutes. More exciting is the potential to reduce the levels of anti-nutrients. Limiting or eliminating the levels of trypsin inhibitor in soybeans for example, would have a major effect on monogastric nutrition. Likewise eliminating phytic acid and/or replacing this with a soluble storage phosphate in the plant, would be welcomed by nutritionists and environmentalists. Eliminating the levels of these 'toxins' may also be more acceptable examples of genetically modified organisms (GMOs) for the consumer. A major challenge facing the feed and broiler industries in using these new ingredients, will be to maintain product identity from the arable field to diet manufacture at the feed mill. Currently soybean meal, as an example, is a single commodity and mill managers are going to be less than enthusiastic when confronted with perhaps 4 or 6 'varieties' bioengineered for various reasons. Bin space is usually a limiting factor at most mills, since these occupy the most space in the physical mill structure.

Some type of HACCP program will become mandatory at feed mills and this will extend from concern over residue of pharmaceutical products through to microbial control. Undoubtedly the microbial status of animal products in general is going to be the single largest factor influencing the success of future production systems. Feed is but one source of such potential contamination, and contrary to popular belief, elimination of meat meal from the formulation is no guarantee of producing feed devoid of microbes pathogenic to birds or humans. It seems obvious that our grains and vegetable proteins are subject to microbial contamination prior to, or in storage at, the feed mills. Few important microbes can withstand feed treatment at 80°C, and so the trend to higher pelleting temperatures. However, recontamination following pelleting is still a major problem, and the use of organic acids/formaldehyde treatments etc. may become more popular to maintain 'clean' feed delivered to the broiler's feed trough.

Disease control

Birds are remarkably healthy considering modern flock sizes and that around 95% of chicks placed, realize their genetic potential. Average mortality is around 3-4% for males and 2-3% for females, depending upon age of marketing. It is doubtful if any other land-based farming operation could manage so successfully, such large numbers of animals within confinement facilities. Our current success is due to genetic selection, availability of efficacious vaccines and antibiotics and a growing awareness of the importance of biosecurity and general farm hygiene.

Current production systems rely on feed-borne antibiotics and growth promoters. With current growth rates of broiler chickens, the classical effects of growth promoters are less easy to quantify. However, most of these compounds are efficacious against Clostridial infection and without them, it is impossible to always control necrotic enteritis and associated outbreaks of coccidiosis. However, it seems as though we are destined to routinely use less of these pharmaceutical products, and while they may be available on prescription for treatment use, alternatives are a fruitful area of research and development. Probiotics and prebiotics seem logical alternatives to antibiotics and growth promoters, and the key to their use is very early dosing of the bird. I think that treatment of chicks on arrival at the farm will, in fact, be too late to prevent colonization of pathogens. This leaves the hatchery as the most logical site for treatment. It is conceivable that treating chicks in their delivery boxes, much as happens with spray vaccines, may also be too late for beneficial live bacteria to become established in the gut. In the future, I think we will see treatment in the hatchers or even at 18d of incubation with incorporation into the Marek's vaccine.

Conclusions

Broiler production systems will increasingly revolve around 'controlled environment' housing with corn and soybean as the basis of our nutritional programs. There will be more emphasis on meeting consumer demands, and this will be accommodated with various value-added meat products. Production will likely be less reliant on antibiotics, growth promoters and anti-coccidials, although this will vary between regions. Microbial status of poultry products will continue to receive much attention, and all segments of the industry will have to work at controlling contamination. In addition, waste from rejected end products (downgraded carcasses etc.) and manure will have to be considered in a situation where concerns for the environment are increasing, and where needs for supplies of 'clean' water for human use are critical.

Increasing emphasis on the inter-relationship between genetic potential, feed and health as well as the need to limit pathogens in the human food chain means that understanding these factors will become increasingly important. Reduced reliance on chemicals and drugs in regions such as Europe will result in an increased reliance on the animals' own natural defences to disease and the exploitation of new methods to ensure genetic growth potential is attained in a cost-effective manner.

Reference

Carte, I.F. (1986) Genetic economics of chicken meat production. In: *Proceedings 3rd Wld Congr. Genetics Appl. Livestock Prod.* **10**: 228-235.

Early gut development: the interaction between feed, gut health and immunity

David Sklan

Faculty of Agriculture, Hebrew University, Rehovot, Israel

Introduction

The following paper examines the morphological development of the gut, its hydrolytic and absorptive capacity, development of microbial populations and the development of an immune system responding to the contents of the gastrointestinal tract.

Gastrointestinal development

Gross development

As incubation progresses embryonic small intestinal weight increases at a much greater rate than body weight close to hatching. During the last three days of incubation the ratio of small intestinal weight to body weight increases from approximately 1% on day 17 of incubation, to 3.5% at hatch. The morphology of the small intestine also changes rapidly with villi developing in at least three phases, with different sized villi found at hatch (Uni et al,et al., 2003).

In the immediate post-hatch period intense changes occur in the small intestines of chicks, as they continue to increase in weight more rapidly then the whole body mass. This rapid relative growth of the small intestines is maximal at 6-8 d in the turkey poult and at 6-10 d in the broiler chick. In contrast, other digestive tract organs such as gizzard and pancreas do not show parallel-enhanced changes in relative size (Uni et al., 1999). The preferential early growth of the small intestine occurs both in the presence and in absence of feed although in the absence of exogenous feed both absolute and relative growth is lower (Noy and Sklan, 1999). In the 'held' bird the substrates for this growth apparently originate from the yolk indicating the high priority for intestinal growth post-hatch. Temporal increases in intestinal weight and length are not identical

9

in the different segments, with the duodenum showing earlier rapid growth then the jejunum and ileum (Uni et al., 1999).

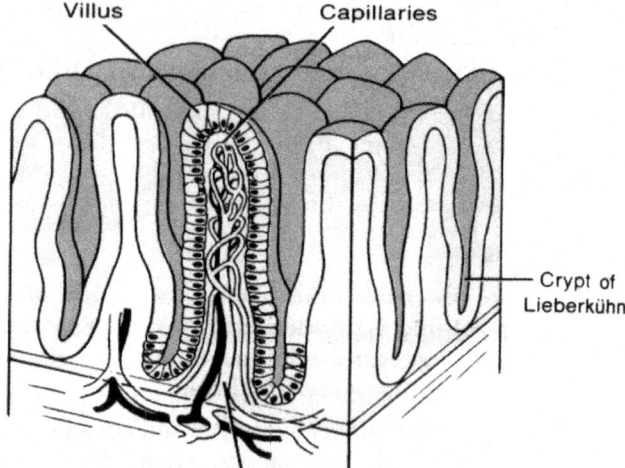

Figure 1.
Cross section of gut wall.

Yolk utilisation

During most of embryonic development in birds yolk is the supplier of nutrients, with the remaining yolk internalized into the abdominal cavity during the last days of incubation (4 , 5). At this time the yolk sac comprises approximately 50% lipids (mainly acylglycerides) and 50% protein. During embryonic development and through hatch, yolk lipids are directly transported to the circulation by endocytosis (Lambson, 1970). However, after internalization close to hatch, yolk is also transported through the yolk stalk to the small intestine (Esteban et al., 1991). Thus two routes of yolk utilization are available (Noy et al., 1996). At hatch the yolk sac is 15-25% of the body weight of chicks and poults and in the immediate post-hatch period yolk is utilized for maintenance and for intestinal growth (Noy and Sklan, 1999), while the birds make the transition from utilizing energy supplied by the endogenous nutrients from the yolk to intestinal utilization of exogenous carbohydrate rich feed. Access to nutrients accelerates the rate of yolk utilization and initiates growth some 24 h post-ingestion and early access to feed results in more rapid intestinal development in the immediate post-hatch period (Sklan, 2001).

Morphological development

At hatch small intestinal enterocytes are round and immediately post-hatch these cells increase rapidly in length and develop a pronounced polarity and defined brush border. At hatch the small intestinal villi are relatively small and in the inter-villus spaces few crypts are detectable. However, within hours of hatching, crypts begin to form and become well defined by 2-3 d. The number of cells per crypt increases rapidly in the 48 h post-hatch in the fed chick and the rate of growth begins decreasing after 48 h (Geyra et al., 2001a). In parallel the number of crypts and their complexity increases rapidly after hatching and this also reaches a plateau after 48-72 h post-hatch. Patterns of crypt development differ between intestinal segments with the duodenum and jejunum continuing to develop after the ileum has reached a constant number of crypts per villus (Geyra et al., 2001a).

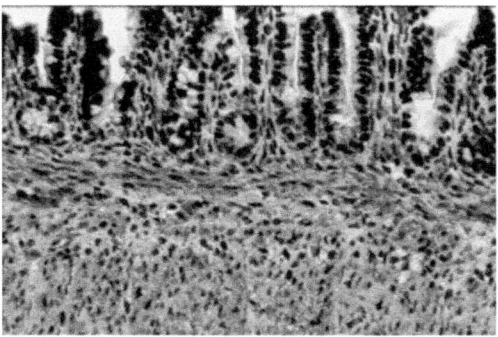

2 hours post hatch

Figure 2.
Crypt structural changes post hatch.

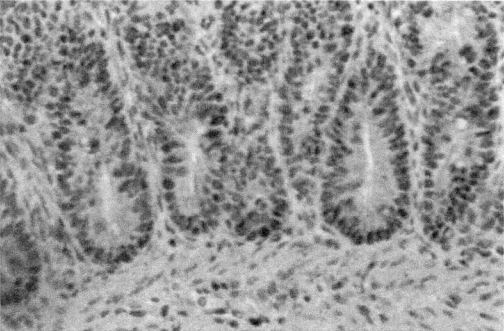

72 hours post hatch

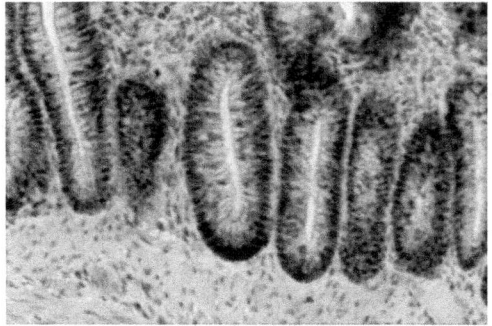

168 hours post hatch

Measurements of the small intestinal mucosa indicates that villus height increases twofold in the 48 h post-hatch and reached a plateau at 6-8 d in the duodenum and after 10 d or more in the jejunum and ileum in chicks. The width of the villi increases only slightly; hence the expansion in surface area tends to be parallel to changes in villus height. Thus total segment surface area increases in all segments in parallel until 3 d post-hatch after which the jejunal surface area continues to enlarge more rapidly then that of the duodenum and ileum. With the growth of the villus the number of enterocytes per villus also multiplies (Geyra et al., 2001a).

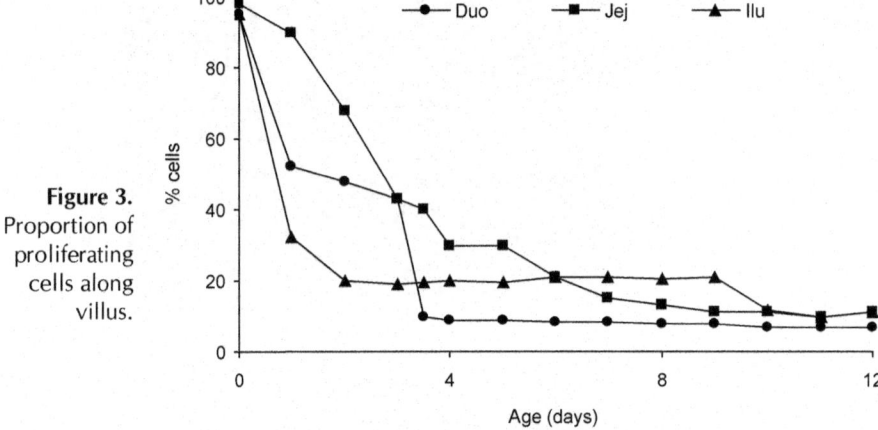

Figure 3. Proportion of proliferating cells along villus.

In both chicks and poults at hatch all small intestinal enterocytes are proliferating. With time the proportions of proliferating cells decreases rapidly, reaching approximately 50% in the crypts after 24-48 h. Along the villus the proportion of proliferating enterocytes reduces quickly at first and then more slowly reaching 6-15% by 10 d post-hatch. Lack of access to feed increases the proportion of proliferating enterocytes both in the crypts and along the villus (Geyra et al., 2001a; 2001b).

Enterocytes migrate from the crypts up the villus until they are exfoliated into the lumen. It is not possible to measure this process before 48 h post-hatch due to the large proportion of proliferating cells along the villus. However, migration from crypt to villus tip takes approximately 72 h in chicks 4 d post hatch and 96 h in older birds (Geyra et al., 2001a; Uni et al., 1998).

The number of goblet cells per villus increases as the villi grows, but the proportion of goblet cells remains constant with age. After hatch goblet cells containing neutral mucin multiply, resulting in

D. Sklan

similar proportions of cells producing both acid and neutral mucin by day 7 post-hatch (Uni et al., 2003).

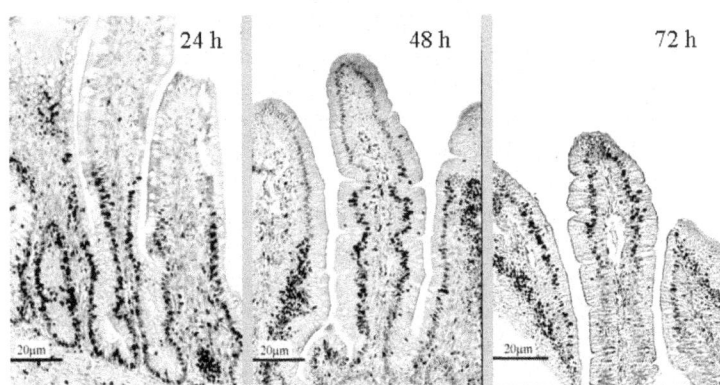

Figure 4. Changes in enterocyte mobility with bird age.

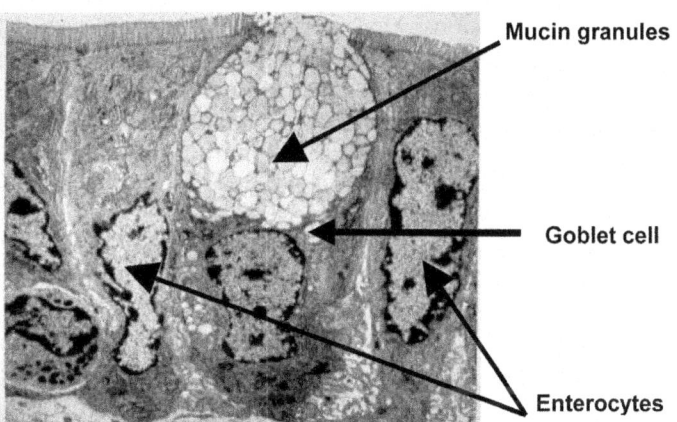

Figure 5. Micrograph of goblet cells within broiler gut wall.

The effect of holding poultry without feed on the morphological development in different intestinal segments in the post-hatch chick has been examined (Geyra et al., 2001b) along with the effect of deutectomy (Uni et al., 1998). Effects of both these treatments on villus surface area are somewhat similar and are regionally dependent. In the duodenum, villus surface area is initially depressed in the absence of feed but reaches values close to those of fed chicks after 4 d, whereas in the jejunum villus surface area is still lower after 9 d. In the ileum no significant effects have been found. Both the number of cells per crypt and the number of crypts per villus are initially decreased by lack of access to feed, although feeding reverses this by 8 d of age. Electron microscopy studies have indicated that 'held' birds show changes in the structure of the micro-villi. In the post-hatch chick recovery of the intestine from lack of access to food for 48 h seems to be relatively complete with the growth rate (but not body weight) of 'held' chicks similar to controls after 6-8 d, and

13

of deutectomised chicks after 8-10 d (Uni et al., 1998; Akiba and Murakami, 1995).

Thus the extensive changes in the morphological development of the small intestines close to hatch include the differentiation of enterocytes and crypt definition as well as enlargement of the intestinal absorptive surface many-fold. These intensive changes are apparently sensitive to perturbations in nutrient supply.

Chicken gut associated lymphoid tissue

Gut associated lymphoid tissue (GALT), a component of the mucosal immune system, has evolved to provide protection against pathogens encountered by the gut. In chickens, GALT is responsible for inducing immune responses against bacterial, viral and parasitic enteric (i.e. introduced via the digestive tract) antigens (Muir et al., 2000; Kajiwara et al., 2003; Yasuda et al., 2002) as well as responses to innocuous antigens (Klipper et al., 2000). The avian GALT contains unique lymphoid structures such as the bursa of Fabricius, caecal tonsils (CT) and Meckel's diverticulum as well as Peyer's patches (PP), intraepithelial lymphocytes (IEL) and scattered immune cells residing in the intestinal lamina propria (Lillehoj and Trout, 1996). As chickens do not have other peripheral encapsulated lymph nodes, GALT lymphoid structures serve as major secondary lymphoid organs (Muir et al., 2000; Gallego et al., 1995; Sayegh et al., 2000; Olah et al., 2003) emphasizing the importance of the avian GALT in protection of birds.

Establishment of immune competence in the avian GALT

Age-related changes in GALT of chickens have been determined and these include changes in composition of T and B lymphocyte populations (Lillehoj, 1993; Yamamoto et al., 1977), innate cell populations (Olah and Glick, 1984) anatomical and morphological changes including enlargement of the bursa and its involution in adulthood, appearance of CT and PP (Gomez et al., 1998) and maturation of the response to enteric pathogens (Lillehoj and Trout, 1996; Befus et al., 1980). Many studies have examined the cellular and functional changes of the avian GALT due to pathogenic challenge (Lillehoj and Trout, 1996; Befus et al., 1980), however, there is less information describing the development and immunological function of the avian GALT in the immediate post-hatch period. This appears to be critical for the chick's survival immediately after hatch, for it is immediately exposed to a wide variety of bacteria.

Population dynamics of intestinal lymphocytes and the temporal development of lymphocyte functions have been studied in broiler chicks during the first 2 weeks post-hatch. Gut-associated lymphoid tissue contains functionally immature T and B-lymphocytes at hatch, and that function is attained during the first 2 weeks of life as demonstrated by mRNA expression of cytokines ChIL-2 and ChIFNγ. Functional maturation occurs in two stages: the first during the 1-7 d post-hatch, and the second during the 8-14 d, which is also accompanied by an increase in lymphocyte population, as determined by expression of antigen receptor genes. In the intestinal milieu, mature cellular immune responses are a prerequisite for humoral responses. Hence, the lack of antibody response in young chicks is primarily due to immaturity of T lymphocytes (Bar-Shira et al., 2003).

One important stimulator of intestinal development in the hatchling is physical exposure to feed, as feed deprivation delays the onset of gut development. As delayed access to feed impairs intestinal development, and intestinal development occurs in concert with that of GALT, effects of short term feed deprivation on GALT development in broiler hatchlings have been examined. These studies determined antibody production, distribution of lymphocytes and expression of lymphocyte specific genes. The findings showed that while development of GALT in the foregut was only slightly and temporarily impeded by feed deprivation, GALT development in the hindgut was severely impaired during the first 35 days of life: Systemic and intestinal antibody responses following rectal immunization to antigen were lower, development of lymphocyte populations in the cloacal bursa was reduced, colonization of the hindgut (caecum and colon) by lymphocytes was reduced and expression of IL-2 mRNA in hindgut lymphocytes was delayed (Bar-Shira et al., 2004). Such findings emphasize the crucial relationship between correct feeding and immune system development.

Development of digestive and absorptive function

Pancreatic enzyme secretions

Intestinal digestion of both yolk and ingested feed from macromolecules to smaller units is affected in the small intestines by enzymes secreted from the pancreas. Marchaim and Kulka (1967) indicated that pancreatic enzymes are present in the small intestines in the late embryonic stages. Determinations of total luminal activities of pancreatic enzymes soon after hatch indicate increases in trypsin, amylase and lipase activities which are correlated with changes in both intestinal and body weights. Chicks without access to feed show little change in trypsin and amylase activities, which increase only after feed consumption (Noy and Sklan, 1999; 2001; Sklan and Noy, 2000; Noy et al., 2001). Determinations of luminal activities of some pancreatic enzymes from 4 d post-hatch using non-absorbed markers indicated increases in secretion of trypsin, amylase and lipase with age (Noy and Sklan, 1995) but not per g feed intake (Uni et al., 1995). It should be noted that secretion of these enzymes exhibit different patterns with development. Lipase activity in the intestine is found even before ingestion of feed, as it is required for hydrolyzing yolk triglycerides (Noy and Sklan, 1998), and (following feed intake) increases in the activity of this enzyme were less dramatic and later then those observed for trypsin and amylase (35,37). However, in fed birds intestinal pancreatic enzymatic activities were correlated both with body weight and intestinal weight (Sklan and Noy, 2001). These findings suggest that feed intake triggers secretion of pancreatic enzymes which are then secreted at relatively constant amounts per feed intake as the chick grows.

Figure 6.
Changes in pancreatic enzyme activities from 0-8d in fed and starved broilers.

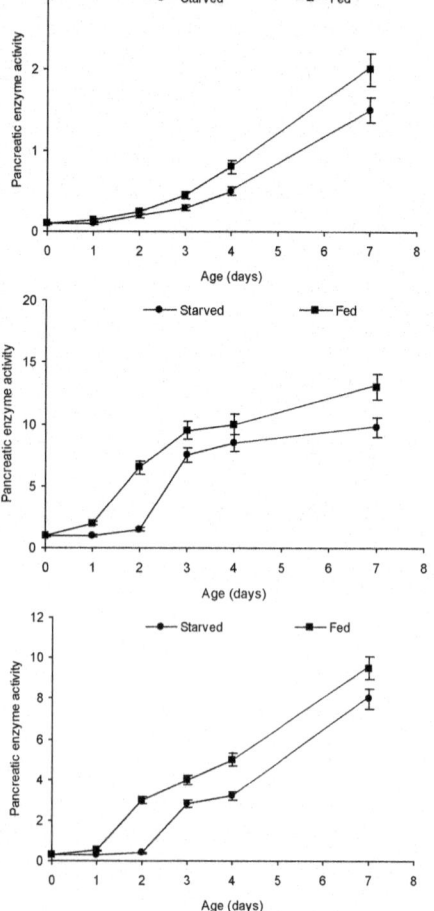

In parallel to the increased pancreatic enzyme secretions the daily secretion of total N and bile acids to the duodenum have been determined from 4 d post-hatch using non-absorbed markers. These increased with both body weight and intestinal weight and when calculated per feed intake showed little change with time.

Mucosal enzyme and transporter activities

In addition to luminal digestion of feed-derived macromolecules, the final stages of hydrolysis are performed by membrane-anchored enzymes at the brush border. These include sucrase-isomaltase, peptidases and phosphatases (Semenza, 1986). Compared to mammals (Aumaitre and Corring, 1978), chickens and poults have high capability to degrade disaccharides in the mucosa immediately post-hatch via the sucrase-maltase enzyme complex. Sucrase-maltase expression increases rapidly just before hatch and continues increasing post-hatch (Smirnov and Sklan, 2003; Sklan et al., 2003). Disaccharides activity per g tissue is lower in the duodenum and higher in jejunal and ileal segments in birds and mammals (Nunez et al., 1996), which is intriguing as they have not been exposed to any carbohydrates before hatching. Expression of the major glucose transporter, SGLT1, increases 2 d pre-hatch and continues to increase post-hatch (Sklan et al., 2003) as does aminopeptidase activity (Uni et al., 2003). In comparison alkaline phosphatase activity changes little with time in the duodenum and jejunum. Thus mucosal enzymes have different developmental timetables which may influence digestion in post-hatch birds. The differences in activities between intestinal regions in the poult are more pronounced than in the chick (Uni et al., 1999).

The mucosal enzyme activity per mass of intestine is closely correlated with the number of enterocytes per villus in all regions of the intestine after 2 d of age, suggesting that that the amount of enzyme activity expressed per enterocyte does not change greatly with age. Calculation of the total mucosal enzyme activity on a regional basis has yielded activity curves for disaccharidases, ε-glutamyl transferase and alkaline phosphatase that are shown to increase curvilinearly with age. Regional activity of mucosal enzymes is related to the digestive capacity in the specific intestinal region.

Basolateral enzyme activities

Most glucose and amino acids are moved into the enterocyte via sodium-dependent transporters, however, for absorption to occur, sodium is required in the lumen and once absorbed must be removed from the enterocytes to maintain ionic equilibrium.

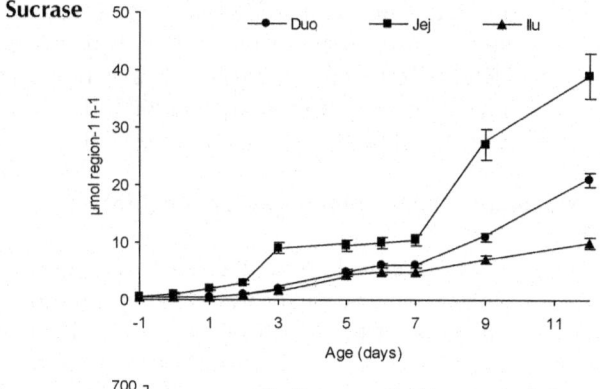

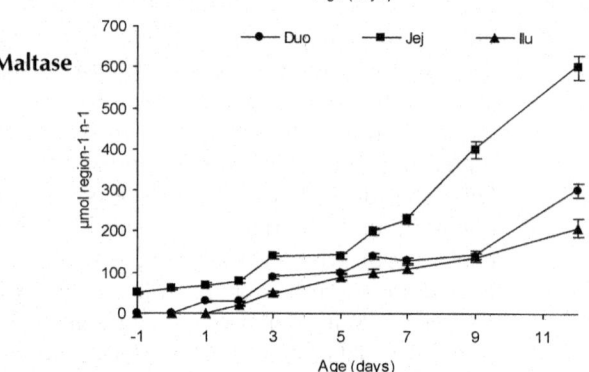

Figure 7.
Development
of brush border
enzyme activity
over time from
different gut
regions.

Sodium transport occurs via the Na-K-ATPase which is located on the enterocyte basolateral membrane; activity of this enzyme reflects total uptake activity of nutrients (Sklan and Noy, 2001). In the post-hatch days the Na-K-ATPase activity increases rapidly in the chick and activities are highly correlated with body weight changes. For higher uptake of nutrients the absorptive activity of the intestine increases and these nutrients then provide the precursors required for the synthesis of body components. Highly significant correlations suggest that mucosal enzyme activity plays a rate-determining role in providing the substrates for growth (Uni et al., 1998).

Mucin production

Mucus is secreted by the goblet cells throughout the gastrointestinal tract and forms a gel adherent to the mucosal surface (Forstner and Forstner, 1994). This layer acts as a barrier between the luminal contents and the absorptive system of the intestine and protects the mucosal surface from exogenous or endogenous luminal irritants such as laxatives (Yagi et al., 1990) or bile salts (Teem and Phillips, 1972) and lumen bacteria. Changes in the properties of this barrier alter absorption of both dietary and endogenous macromolecules and ions (Satchithanandam et al., 1990; Quarterman, 1987). Mucin secreting cells have been observed in the small intestine of the chick at pipping and at this time only acid mucins were observed. After hatch the proportion of goblet cells increases and both acid and neutral mucins are found. The role of mucin in absorption and in protection against pathogens and the age at which the mucin layer acts as a functional barrier are not yet fully understood.

Intestinal uptake

Intestinal uptake capacity has been examined *in vitro*, in situ and in vivo and indirectly in young birds. Studies in vitro indicated that per g intestine, uptake of glucose and methionine increased somewhat after hatch in chicks (Noy et al., 1996; Shehata et al., 1984) and poults between hatch and 7 d old (Noy and Sklan, 1998). *In situ* studies in post-hatch birds with buffered solutions indicated little change in uptake per g small intestine with age (Sklan and Noy, 2001). However, there are distinct differences close to hatch between uptake from buffered solutions in vitro and in situ as compared to yolk-containing solutions (Sklan and Noy, 2001). Absorption of glucose or methionine from yolk-containing solutions was generally only 20-35% of uptake from buffered medium. This has been attributed in part to the hydrophobic nature of yolk and also to the low luminal concentrations of sodium which is required for full activity of the sodium-glucose and sodium-amino acid co-transporters close to hatch (Noy and Sklan, 1999).

In vivo, non-absorbed marker determinations immediately post-hatch have indicated that uptake of glucose and methionine is relatively low, increasing by 4 d post-hatch (Noy and Sklan, 1999). This low uptake of hydrophilic components has been confirmed by TME measurements indicating low availability of carbohydrates and proteins close to hatch. Availability of both increases with age, reaching adult values by 10 d (Sulistiyanto et al., 1999). In contrast lipids are efficiently taken up from the hydrophobic yolk-rich medium (Noy and Sklan, 1999).

Overall absorption studies from 4 d using non-absorbed marker techniques revealed that starch and fatty acids were more than 85% absorbed after 4 d, whereas protein digestion increased from 70-78% at 4 d to 85% by 14 d (Noy and Sklan, 1995; Uni et al., 1996). Thus although uptake of hydrophilic molecules is not complete close to hatch, absorption reaches high levels by 10 d.

19

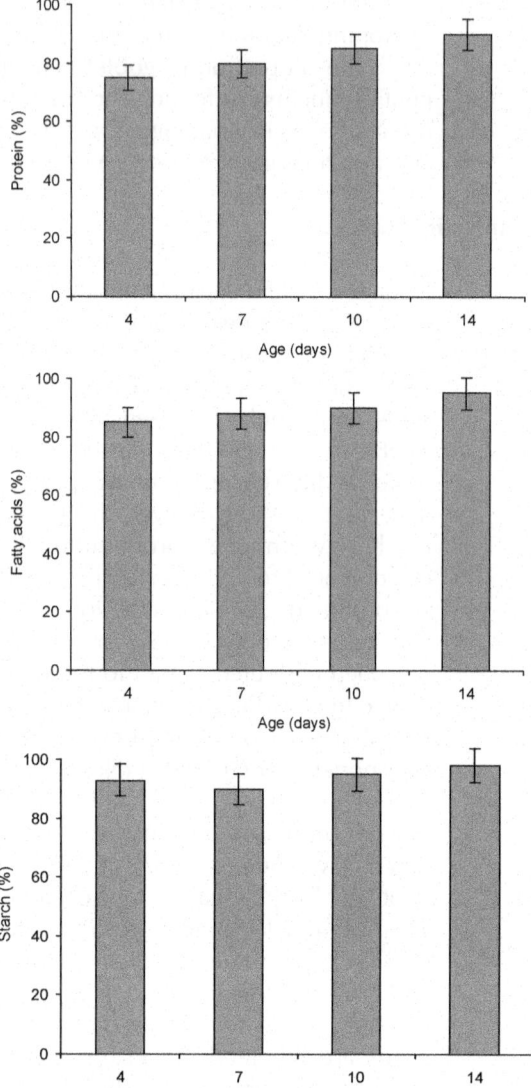

Figure 8.
Ileal absorption
of protein (N),
fatty acids (FA)
and starch in
4-14 d broiler
chicks.

Development of gut microflora

A diverse micro-biota develops throughout the gastrointestinal tract
and is most extensive in the caeca (Barnes, 1972; Barnes et al.,
1972; Mead, 1997; Mead and Adams, 1975). The gut microflora
influences health and intestinal responses of host animals in many
ways which will be discussed below (Mead, 1997 ; van der Wielen

et al., 2002; Nurmi and Rantala, 1973; Vispo and Karasov, 1997). In poultry, the absence of normal microflora in the caeca has been considered to be a major factor in the susceptibility of chicks to bacterial infection (Barrow, 1992). Although the alimentary tract of the newly hatched chick is usually sterile, organisms rapidly gain access from the surrounding environment. Large numbers of anaerobic bacteria, capable of decomposing uric acid comprise the caecal flora of chicks 3 to 6 h after hatching (Mead et al., 1975). During the first 2 to 4 d post-hatch Streptococci and Enterobacteria colonize the small intestine and caecum. After the first week Lactobacillus predominate in the small intestine and the caecum is colonized mainly by obligate anaerobes (*E. coli* and Bacteroides) with lower numbers of facultative aerobes (Mead and Adams, 1975; Lev and Briggs, 1956).

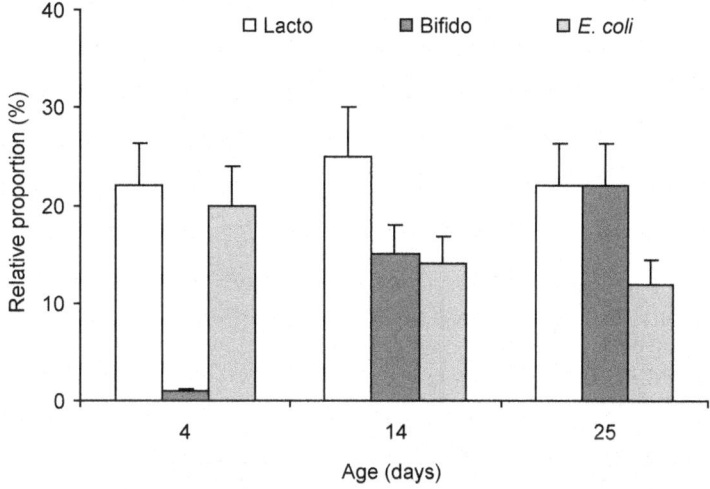

Figure 9. Changes in proportions of caecal bacterial populations with age in the broiler.

A typical microflora of adult birds in the small intestine is established within 2 weeks, however, it was found that the adult caecal flora (mainly obligate anaerobes) takes up to 30 d to develop, At that age Bifidobacteria and Bacteroides predominate (Barnes et al., 1972) and the adult microflora comprises a biomass of up to 10^{13} cells comprised of several hundreds of species. This flora is not constant and can be altered either through the feed or via the cloaca.

Development of immune competence in the gut

The gut-associated lymphoid system (GALT) is confronted with two types of antigenic molecules: a) innocuous antigens, namely those that are basically nutrients and as such should not evoke immune responses. b) Antigens derived from intestinal or external pathogens that should evoke protective immune responses. Hence, the balance between response and tolerance in the gut is finely tuned and depends to a great deal on the interaction between immune cells and those of the gut parenchyma. In a broad sense any antigenic molecule that is absorbed via enterocytes (intracellular transcytosis) is tolerogenic, whereas any antigenic moiety that penetrates the intestinal lining either via transcellular pathways or via phagocytic lining cells (i.e. M cells) is immunogenic.

In the chicken, the most significant contact with microflora occurs in the distal intestine. This is due to both the presence of hindgut fermentation in the caeca and to the influx of bacteria via the cloaca by means of retrograde peristalsis. The retrograde movement of the cloaca and colon also serves two immunologically relevant functions: a) a means to transport antibodies secreted via the bursal canal and that originate from the bursa of Fabricius and bursal canal lymphoid follicles, and b) sampling external bacteria via the rectum (Friedman et al., 2003).

Figure 10. Development of the bursa in broiler chickens (adapted from Dibner *et al.*, 1998)

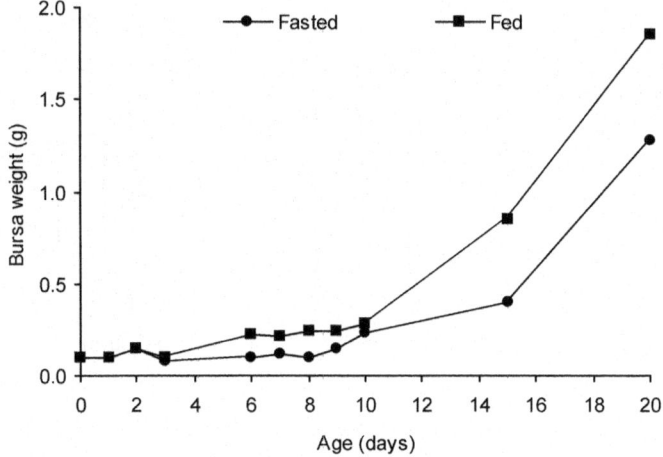

Protection of the gut is achieved by both innate and adaptive means. Conceptually, the best strategy to avoid infection is to prevent binding between pathogen and enterocyte (Sanderson and Walker, 1999). This may be achieved by secreting anti-bacterial substances from innate cells of the epithelial lining (Paneth-like cells of the crypt) or more specifically by secreting neutralizing antibodies into the intestinal lumen. Thus, both non-specific and immunological barriers serve to prevent binding and absorption of pathogenic moieties (Sanderson and Walker, 1999). Neutralizing antibodies are either of IgG, monomeric IgA or dimeric IgA isotypes (Klipper et al., 2000; Mestecky et al., 1999). IgG and monomeric IgA are secreted into the gut via bile in the foregut or via the bursal canal in the hindgut (Klipper et al., 2000). Plasma cells secreting IgC or dimeric IgA reside in the intestinal wall or elsewhere in the chicken (Sharma, 1991; Fagerland and Arp, 1993), and dimerica IgA is secreted via enterocytes (Mestecky et al., 1999). In this case dimeric IgA, secreted by local plasma cells, is taken up by the polymeric IG receptor located in the basal membrane of enterocytes. IgA is then transported to the apical membrane, and secreted into the intestinal lumen (Muir et al., 2000; Mestecky et al., 1999).

The basis of the developing adaptive immune response is the lymphoid follicle. This unique structure contains naive lymphocytes, both T and B, undergoing differentiation and division in the process of generating effector lymphocytes. Dividing lymphocytes are selected by merit of antigen binding as presented by follicular dendritic cells. Selected cells then differentiate into effectors or memory cells, both of which may migrate to tissues. Primary follicles of this nature are scarce in the small intestines of the chick (Befus et al., 1980) and most primary responses are probably generated in the chick hindgut, bursal canal, bursa of Fabricus and spleen. These primary responses become systemic as locally produced antibody is found in the plasma and effector cells migrate to other parts of gut or chick (spleen, bone marrow etc). Hence, protection of the gut is achieved by generating immune responses in the hindgut and bursal canal followed by systemic dissemination of these responses throughout the gut and bird.

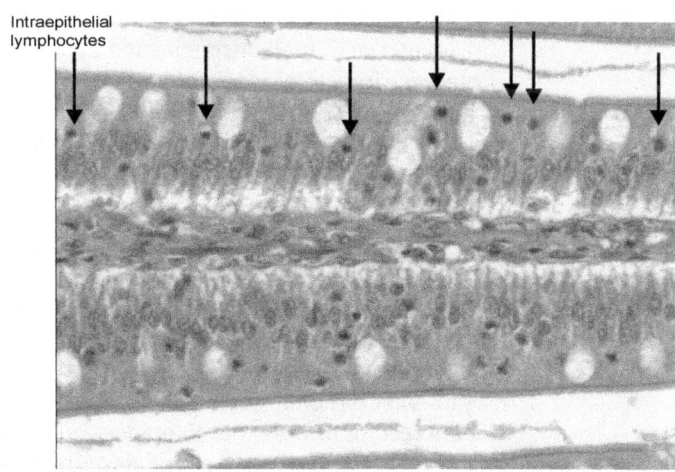

Intraepithelial lymphocytes

Figure 11. Cross section of broiler gut wall showing intraepithelial lymphocytes.

A key issue in the function of the hindgut in generation of immune responses lies in its ability to sample antigen material from the exterior. The evidence supporting this is from studies demonstrating retrograde contractions of the intestinal duct. Previous studies in hatchlings and mature birds have indicated reverse peristalsis of digesta from mid jejunum to duodenum and even gizzard (Noy and Sklan, 1998). Together these studies indicate an avenue for rectally derived external material to reach the immunologically active caeca, and importantly, a pathway fro bursa derived antibodies up to the small intestine (Clench, 1999).

The bursa and bursal canal have a significant role in the generation of gut-protective immune responses. Antigen is actively transported via the bursal canal into the bursal lumen (Befus et al., 1980; Sorvari et al., 1975). Further more, antigen bound by follicular associated epithelium (FAE) (Bockman and Cooper, 1973) can then induce immune responses in both the canal wall and bursal tissue in which both mature T and B-lymphocytes have been demonstrated (Khan and Hashimoto, 1996). Effector plasma cells are observed in connective tissue proximal to FAE, and in the lamina propria of the bursal canal lining (Naukkarinen and Sorvari, 1982). The bursa is enclosed in a capsule of smooth muscle, contractions of which then propel secretions towards the bursal canal, and from there into the cloaca. The secreta can then be transported by the colon via retrograde peristalsis, and distributed to proximal gut sections as indicated above.

The GALT is confronted with both noxious and innocuous antigens. The former lead to immune responses, while the latter should not, and rather be ignored or tolerated. This dichotomy has been demonstrated in several mammalian species where oral protein antigens induce tolerance (oral tolerance) (Friedman et al., 1994). Surprisingly, in the chicken, oral protein antigens delivered in aqueous solutions induce potent immune responses and not oral tolerance (Friedman et al., 1994; Klipper et al., 2000; 2001). Interestingly, the same protein antigens are ignored by the immune system if supplied as solids in the ration (Klipper et al., 2001). These observations were initially made in adult chickens and similar experiments in hatchlings up to day 10 of life showed a brief 3-4 day period in which tolerance may be induced by oral antigen (Klipper et al., 2001). The functional difference in the 4 day old intestine and GALT that allows induction of tolerance rather than response has yet to be determined, but it is interesting to note that tolerance-induction precedes the second wave of lymphoid colonization described above. Thus, as the chick immediately begins to forage, the intestinal immune system is geared towards tolerance, while the subsequent colonization by flora is met with an immunologically more mature GALT programmed for response. Furthermore, maintenance of antigen specific tolerance induced during the 4-day window is dependent upon re-exposure to the tolerising antigen; if such an antigen is denied for 4-6 weeks – tolerance is replaced by oral responses. Presently, it is not known whether oral tolerance is induced in the gut, peripheral or central immune organs.

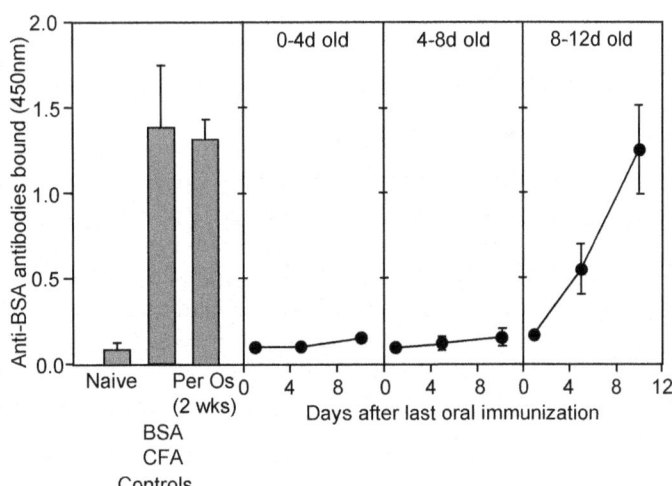

Figure 12. Development of antibody responses to oral antigens in the broiler (Bar-Shira *et al.*, 2003).

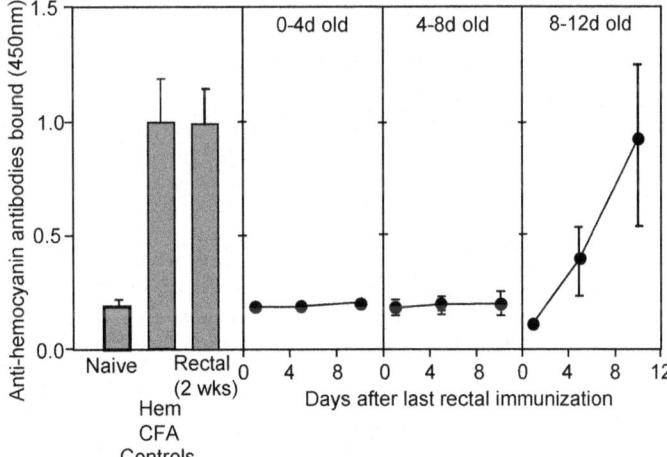

Figure 13. Development of antibody responses to rectal antigens in the broiler (Bar-Shira *et al.*, 2003).

Interrelationships

Many associations between growth and the absorptive processes described above have been elucidated. Body weight is correlated to feed intake, and studies using the intestinal basolateral Na-K-

ATPase activity to estimate uptake have also shown that this was highly correlated with growth. Villus and intestinal segment area in all three intestinal segments in the immediate post-hatch period, and, in addition, both pancreatic enzymatic activities and mucosal segment activities are all correlated with growth (Sklan, 2001). It is more difficult to examine the interrelationships with immune function and microbial populations; however, research is beginning to generate more information which is required to integrate the wide variety of processes occurring in the gut.

Summary

Ingestion of feed in the young chick is accompanied by the development of microbial populations in the gut. Intestinal development after hatch is rapid with increases in hydrolytic and absorptive capacities and immune functions. Early exposure to feed appears to enhance maturation of all of the above functions. Since the GALT is not immediately mature early contact with a hostile environment is more likely to compromise health then later exposure. In addition, early foraging may promote development of immune function by increasing access of hindgut to environmental microflora.

References

Akiba, Y. and Murakami, H. (1995) Partitioning of energy and protein during early growth of broiler chicks and contribution of vitelline residue. *10th European Symposium on Poultry Nutrition*, Antalia, Turkey.

Aumaitre, A. and Corring, T. (1978) Development of digestive enzymes in the piglet from birth to 8 weeks. II. Intestine and intestinal disaccharidases. *Nutrition and Metabolism* **22**: 244-255.

Barnes, E. M. (1972) The avian intestinal flora with particular reference to the possible ecological significance of the caecal anaerobic bacteria. *American Journal of Clinical Nutrition* **25**: 1475-1479.

Barnes, E. M., Mead, G. C., Barnum, D. A. and Harry, E. G. (1972) The intestinal flora of the chicken in the period 2 to 6 weeks of age, with particular reference to the anaerobic bacteria. *British Poultry Science* **13**: 311-326.

Barrow, P. (1992) Probiotic for chickens. In: *Probiotics, the Scientific Basis* Edited by Fuller, R., pp. 225-257. Chapman and Hall, London.

Bar-Shira, E., Sklan, D. and Friedman, A. (2003) Establishment of immune competence in the avian GALT during the immediate post-hatch period. *Developmental and Comparative Immunology* **27**: 147-157.

Bar-Shira, E., Sklan, D. and Friedman, A. (2004) in press.

Befus, A. D., Johnston, N., Leslie, G. A. and Bienenstock, J. (1980) Gut-associated lymphoid tissue in the chicken. I. Morphology, ontogeny, and some functional characteristics of Peyer's patches. *Journal of Immunology* **125**: 2626-2632.

Bockman, D. E. and Cooper, M. D. (1973) Pinocytosis by epithelium associated with lymphoid follicles in the bursa of Fabricius, appendix, and Peyer's patches. An electron microscopic study. *American Journal of Anatomy* **136**: 455-477.

Clench, M. H. (1999) The avian caecum: uptake and motility review. *Journal of Experimental Zoology* **283**: 441-447.

Esteban, S., Moreno, M., Rayo, J. M. and Tur, J. A. (1991) Gastrointestinal emptying in the final days of incubation of the chick embryo. *British Poultry Science* **32**: 279-284.

Fagerland, J. A. and Arp, L. H. (1993) Distribution and quantification of plasma cells, T lymphocyte subsets, and B lymphocytes in bronchus-associated lymphoid tissue of chickens: age-related differences. *Regional Immunology* **5**: 28-36.

Forstner, J. F. and Forstner, G. G. (1994) Gastrointestinal mucus. In: *Physiology of the Gastrointestinal Tract*, 3rd ed. Edited by Johnson Leonard, R., pp. 1255-1284. Raven, New York.

Friedman, A., al-Sabbagh, A., Santos, L. M., Fishman-Lobell, J., Polanski, M., Das, M. P., Koury, S. J. and Weiner, H. L. (1994) Oral tolerance: a biological relevant pathway to generate peripheral tolerance against external and self antigens. *Chemical Immunology* **58**: 259-290.

Friedman, A., Bar Shira, E. and Sklan, D. (2003) Ontogeny of gut associated immune competence in the chick. *Worlds Poultry Science Journal* **59**: 209-219.

Gallego, M., Cacho, E. D. and Bascuas, J. A. (1995) Antigen-binding cells in the Caecal tonsils and Peyer's patches of the chicken after bovine serum albumin administration. *Poultry Science* **74**: 472-479.

Geyra, A., Uni, Z. and Sklan, D. (2001) Enterocyte dynamics and mucosal development in the posthatch chick. *Poultry Science* **80**: 776-782.

Geyra, A., Uni, Z. and Sklan, D. (2001) The effect of fasting at different ages on growth and tissue dynamics in the small intestine of the young chick. *British Journal of Nutrition* **86**: 53-61.

Gomez Del Moral, M., Fonfria, J., Varas, A., Jimenez, E., Moreno, J. and Zapata, A. G. (1998) Appearance and development of lymphoid cells in the chicken (Gallus gallus) caecal tonsil. *Anatomical Record* **250**: 182-189.

Kajiwara, E., Shigeta, A., Horiuchi, H., Matsuda, H. and Furusawa,

S. (2003) Development of Peyer's Patch and Caecal Tonsil in Gut-Associated Lymphoid Tissues in the Chicken Embryo. *Journal of Veterinary Medical Science* **65**: 607-614.

Khan, M. Z. and Hashimoto, Y. (1996) An immuno-histochemical analysis of T-cell subsets in the chicken bursa of Fabricius during postnatal stages of development. *Journal of Veterinary Medical Science* **58**: 1231-1234.

Klipper, E., Sklan, D. and Friedman, A. (2000) Immune response of chickens to dietary protein antigens. *Veterinary Immunology and Immunopathology* **74**: 209-223.

Klipper, E., Sklan, D. and Friedman, A. (2001) Response, tolerance and ignorance following oral exposure to a single protein antigen in *Gallus domesticus*. *Vaccine* **19**: 2890-2897.

Lambson, R. O. (1970) An electron microscopic study of the entodermal cells of the yolk sac of the chick during incubation and after hatching. *American Journal of Anatomy* **129**: 1-19.

Lev, M. and Briggs, C. A. E. (1956) The gut flora of the chicks. 1. The flora of newly hatched chicks. *Journal of Applied Bacteriology* **19**: 36-38.

Lillehoj, H. S. (1993) Avian gut-associated immune system: implication in coccidial vaccine development. *Poultry Science* **72**: 1306-1311.

Lillehoj, H. S. and Trout, J. M. (1996) Avian gut-associated lymphoid tissues and intestinal immune responses to Eimeria parasites. *Clinical Microbiology Reviews* **9**: 349-360.

Marchaim, U. and Kulka, R. G. (1967) The non-parallel increase of amylase chymotrypsinogen and procarboxypeptidase in the developing chick pancreas. *Biochimica et Biophysica Acta* **146**: 553-559.

Mead, G. C. (1997) Bacteria in the gastrointestinal tract of birds. In: *Gastrointestinal Microbiology. 2. Gastrointestinal Microbes and Host interactions* Edited by Mackie, R. J., White, B. A. and Isaacson, R. E., pp. 216-240. Chapman and Hall, New York.

Mead, G. C. and Adams, B. W. (1975) Some observations on the caecal microflora of the chick during the first two weeks of life. *British Poultry Science* **16**: 169-176.

Mestecky, J., Moro, I. and Underdown, B. J. (1999) Mucosal Immunoglobulins. In: *Mucosal Immunology*, Second edition edited by Ogra, P. L., Mestecky, J., Lamm, M. E., Strober, W., Bienenstock, J. and McGhee, J. R. pp. 133-152. Academic Press, London.

Muir, W. I., Bryden, W. L. and Husband, A. J. (2000) Immunity, vaccination and the avian intestinal tract. *Developmental and Comparative Immunology* **24**: 325-342.

Naukkarinen, A. and Sorvari, T. E. (1982) Morphological and histochemical characterization of the medullary cells in the bursal follicles of the chicken. Acta Pathologica et Microbiologica Scandinavica. Section C, *Immunology* **90**: 193-199.

Noble, R. and Ogunyemi, D. (1989) Lipid changes in the residual yolk and liver of the chick immediately after hatching. *Biology of the Neonate* **56**: 228-236.

Noy, Y. and Sklan, D. (1995) Digestion and absorption in the young chick. *Poultry Science* **74**: 366-373.

Noy, Y. and Sklan, D. (1998) Yolk utilisation in the newly hatched poult. *British Poultry Science* **39**: 446-451.

Noy, Y. and Sklan, D. (1999) Energy utilization in newly hatched chicks. *Poultry Science* **78**: 1750-1756.

Noy, Y. and Sklan, D. (2001) Yolk and exogenous feed utilization in the posthatch chick. *Poultry Science* **80**: 1490-1495.

Noy, Y., Geyra, A. and Sklan, D. (2001) The effect of early feeding on growth and small intestinal development in the posthatch poult. *Poultry Science* **80**: 912-919.

Noy, Y., Uni, Z. and Sklan, D. (1996) Routes of Yolk Utilization in the Newly-Hatched Chick. *British Poultry Science* **37**: 987-996.

Nunez, M. C., Bueno, J. D., Ayudarte, M. V., Almendros, A., Rios, A., Suarez, M. D. and Gil, A. (1996) Dietary restriction induces biochemical and morphometric changes in the small intestine of nursing piglets. *Journal of Nutrition* **126**: 933-944.

Nurmi, E. and Rantala, M. (1973) New aspects of Salmonella infection in broiler production. *Nature* **241**: 210-211.

Olah, I. and Glick, B. (1984) Meckel's diverticulum. I. Extramedullary myelopoiesis in the yolk sac of hatched chickens (Gallus domesticus). *Anatomical Record* **208**: 243-252.

Olah, I., Nagy, N., Magyar, A. and Palya, V. (2003) Esophageal tonsil: a novel gut-associated lymphoid organ. *Poultry Science* **82**: 767-770.

Quarterman, J. (1987) Metal absorption and the intestinal mucus layer. *Digestion* **37**: 1-9.

Romanoff, A. (1960) *The Avian Embryo*. Macmillan, New York.

Sanderson, I. R. and Walker, W. A. (1999) Mucosal barrier: an overview. In: *Mucosal Immunology*, Second edition edited by Ogra, P. L., Mestecky, J., Lamm, M. E., Strober, W., Bienenstock, J. and McGhee, J. R. pp. 5-18. Academic Press, London.

Satchithanandam, S., Vargofcak-Apker, M., Calvert, R. J., Leeds, A. R. and Cassidy, M. M. (1990) Alteration of gastrointestinal mucin by fiber feeding in rats. *Journal of Nutrition* **120**: 1179-1184.

Sayegh, C. E., Demaries, S. L., Pike, K. A., Friedman, J. E. and Ratcliffe, M. J. (2000) The chicken B-cell receptor complex and its role in avian B-cell development. *Immunological Reviews* **175**: 187-200.

Semenza, G. (1986) Anchoring and biosynthesis of stalked brush border membrane proteins: glycosidases and peptidases of enterocytes and renal tubuli. *Annual Review of Cell Biology* **2**: 255-313.

Sharma, J. M. (1991) Overview of the avian immune system. *Veterinary Immunology and Immunopathology* **30**: 13-17.

Shehata, A. T., Lerner, J. and Miller, D. S. (1984) Development of nutrient transport systems in chick jejunum. *American Journal of Physiology* **246**: G101-107.

Sklan, D. (2001) Development of the digestive tract of poultry. *World's Poultry Science Journal* **57**: 415-428.

Sklan, D. and Noy, Y. (2000) Hydrolysis and absorption in the small intestines of posthatch chicks. *Poultry Science* **79**: 1306-1310.

Sklan, D., Geyra, A., Tako, E., Gal-Gerber, O. and Uni, Z. (2003) Ontogeny of brush border carbohydrate digestion and uptake in the chick. *British Journal of Nutrition* **89**: 747-753.

Sorvari, R. and Sorvari, T. E. (1978) Bursal fabricii as a peripheral lymphoid organ. Transport of various materials from the anal lips to the bursal lymphoid follicles with reference to its immunological importance. *Immunology* **32**: 499-505.

Sorvari, R., Naukkarinen, A. and Sorvari, T. E. (1977) Anal sucking-like movements in the chicken and chick embryo followed by the transportation of environmental material to the bursa of Fabricius, caeca and caecal tonsils. *Poultry Science* **56**: 1426-1429.

Sorvari, T., Sorvari, R., Ruotsalainen, P., Toivanen, A. and Toivanen, P. (1975) Uptake of environmental antigens by the bursa of Fabricius. *Nature* **253**: 217-219.

Sulistiyanto, B., Akiba, Y. and Sato, K. (1999) Energy utilization of carbohydrate, fat and protein sources in newly hatched broiler chicks. *British Poultry Science* **40**: 653-659.

Teem, M. V. and Phillips, T. E. (1972) Perfusion of the hamster jejunum with conjugated and unconjugated bile acids: inhibition of water absorption and effects on morphology. *Gastroenterology* **62**: 261-267.

Uni, Z., Ganot, S. and Sklan, D. (1998) Posthatch development of mucosal function in the broiler small intestine. *Poultry Science* **77**: 75-82.

Uni, Z., Noy, Y. and Sklan, D. (1995) Posthatch changes in morphology and function of the small intestines in heavy- and light-strain chicks. *Poultry Science* **74**: 1622-1629.

Uni, Z., Noy, Y. and Sklan, D. (1996) Development of the small intestine in heavy and light strain chicks before and after hatching. *British Poultry Science* **37**: 63-71.

Uni, Z., Noy, Y. and Sklan, D. (1999) Posthatch development of small intestinal function in the poult. *Poultry Science* **78**: 215-222.

Uni, Z., Smirnov, A. and Sklan, D. (2003) Pre- and posthatch development of goblet cells in the broiler small intestine: effect of delayed access to feed. *Poultry Science* **82**: 320-327.

Uni, Z., Tako, E., Gal-Garber, O. and Sklan, D. (2003) Morphological, molecular, and functional changes in the chicken small intestine of the late-term embryo. *Poultry Science* **82**: 1747-1754.

van der Wielen, P. W., Keuzenkamp, D. A., Lipman, L. J., van Knapen, F. and Biesterveld, S. (2002) Spatial and temporal variation of the intestinal bacterial community in commercially raised broiler chickens during growth. *Microbial Ecology* **44**: 286-293.

Vispo, c. and Karasov, W. H. (1997) The interaction of avian gut microbes and their host: an elusive symbiosis. In: *Gastrointestinal Microbiology. 1. Gastrointestinal Ecosystem and Fermentations*. Edited by Mackie, R. J. and White, B. A, pp. 116-155. Chapman and Hall, New York.

Yagi, T., Miyawaki, Y., Nishikawa, A., Horiyama, S., Yamuchi, K. and Kuwano, S. (1990) Prostaglandin E2-mediated stimulation of mucus synthesis and secretion rhenin anthone, the active metabolite of sennosides A and B in mouse colon. *Journal of Pharmacy and Pharmacology* **42**: 542-545.

Yamamoto, H., Watanabe, H. and Mikami, T. (1977) Distribution of immunoglobulin and secretory component containing cells in chickens. *American Journal of Veterinary Research* **38**: 1227-1230.

Yasuda, M., Tanaka, S., Arakawa, H., Taura, Y., Yokomizo, Y. and Ekino, S. (2002) A comparative study of gut-associated lymphoid tissue in calf and chicken. *Anatomical Record* **266**: 207-217.

Interaction of nutrition with intestinal microbial communities

Ortwin Simon, Wilfried Vahjen and David Taras
Institute of Animal Nutrition, Faculty of Veterinary Medicine, Free University of Berlin, Germany

Introduction

When focussing on bacteria, the overall process of digestion in the gastrointestinal tract of monogastric animals is commonly described as occurring in either the small intestine or the hindgut. For example, catalytic enzyme activity and other factors produced by the host are active in the small intestine, and conversions of remaining nutrients by bacterial activities are restricted to the hindgut. This is true with regard to major nutrient conversions. However, it is known that bacteria are present in the chyme and epithelia along the digestive tract of pigs. The significance of bacterial metabolic activities in precaecal sections is already visible in the small intestine and can be shown by partial degradation of non-starch-polysaccharides (NSP) like pectins, 1-3,1-4 ß-glucans or arabinoxylans; by formation of bacterial metabolic products like lactate and short chain fatty acids as well as by deconjugation of bile acids.

Antibiotics have been used as growth promoters in various species of farm animals for many years. Benefits include reduced frequency of diarrhoea under certain conditions, and beneficial effects on performance parameters such as body weight gain or feed conversion ratio up to approximately 5 per cent. These effects are explained by the modification of intestinal bacterial populations and their interaction with the host animal. They might include interactions with intestinal epithelial tissues (proliferation and apoptosis of epithelial cells, surface coating – mucin formation and secretion, invasions and lesions) and the immune system (response of the lymphocyte population and of formation and secretion of immunoglobulins).

From the above it is obvious that the intestinal microbiota is not only greatly involved in nutrient conversion along the gastrointestinal tract, but may also affect or support animal health. Thus, modifications of intestinal microbial communities may lead to beneficial effects for the animal that are measurable as improvements in animal performance.

The EU will impose a total ban on the use of the 4 remaining in-feed antibiotic growth promoters (AGPs) by January 2006. This has resulted in an even greater emphasis to develop, and investigate the effects of non-pharmaceutical feed ingredients on animal health and performance. Many of these ingredients are often thought to exert their effects through modification of the intestinal microbiota. Among these so-called 'alternatives to antibiotics' are probiotics (micro-organisms), prebiotics (carbohydrates specifically utilised by desired bacteria groups), organic acids and herbs/essential oils.

In this context some studies concerning the effects of diet constituents on intestinal microbial communities in monogastric animals will be discussed.

Characterisation of the intestinal microbiota

Conventional microbiology

Our knowledge concerning intestinal bacterial species was founded by cultural methods, *i.e.* cultivation of samples in selective media, generation of pure cultures and subsequent taxonomic identification of the unknown bacterium. In the late 19th century the practical success of this method for the identification of bacteria has led to the general believe among medical scientists that all bacteria are cultivatable by existing methods. One outcome of this approach was the idea that *Escherichia coli* is the dominating intestinal bacterium, simply because early studies on intestinal microbiology showed highest colony counts for *E. coli*. Today, we know that *E. coli* is only a minor member of intestinal bacterial communities, as improved cultivation media and anaerobic techniques by far exceeded the sensitivity of early studies and enabled isolation and cultivation of a multitude of different species. Nevertheless, microscopic counts of native samples and subsequent colony counts after cultivation may differ by more than 2 $\log_{10}$ units. This shows that cultivation methods have not yet reached their full potential and may never be able to allow growth of all bacteria within a given sample.

The main disadvantages of cultivation are unknown growth requirements or environmental conditions that cannot be reproduced outside the intestine (*i.e.* under *in vitro* conditions). Many intestinal bacteria develop symbiotic relationships with other bacteria, *i.e.* without growth of one partner the other may not be cultivatable. Bacteria living in close proximity to epithelial tissues are also very specialised in terms of nutrient requirements as well as growth behaviour and may take more time to grow on conventional media. For instance, *Helicobacter pylori*, the bacterium responsible for stomach ulcers in humans, was only detected by coincidence, because agar plates were left in the incubator over a holiday weekend, instead of the usual 48 hour incubation period. Most famous for their unculturability are segmented filamentous bacteria that are abundant in the intestine of young animals. These very large, firmly attached bacteria have yet to be isolated as pure cultures, although their function as immune-stimulating agents has already been reported (Meyerholz *et al.*, 2002).

Finally, taxonomic arrangement of bacteria into groups, genera and species is most often carried out by biochemical characterisation, for example, by studies on enzyme activity or metabolite production. Strains within a species sometimes do not follow the biochemical paths of the majority of strains and thus give seemingly erroneous results. Furthermore, genes located on plasmids may be lost during subculture and inadequate culture conditions may lead to the loss of inactive physiological traits.

From the above it can be concluded that conventional microbiology is not the method of choice for the investigation of intestinal bacteria. However, cultivation and growth in pure culture is still the only way to characterise new bacterial strains, because only cell material can be studied for metabolic activities.

Although cultivation has the above-mentioned disadvantages, the results of such methods may provide a crude indication of the main functional groups of intestinal bacteria (Table 1). The stomach of the pig is dominated by Lactobacilli, which also form one of the major functional groups within the small intestine. Together with Enterococci and Streptococci (mainly *S. agalactolyticus*), these lactic acid bacteria dominate the proximal small intestine with lesser amounts of Enterobacteria and other transient bacteria. Gradual changes along the small intestine can be observed within lactic acid bacteria species as well as the occurrence of strict anaerobic bacteria (Bacteroides, Clostridia). In the hindgut strict anaerobes outnumber lactic acid bacteria and other bacteria by factors of 10 to 100.

Molecular microbiology

The use of molecular biology methods has greatly enhanced our knowledge of gastrointestinal bacterial communities. More specifically, ribosomal DNA (rDNA) has been shown to be an excellent marker in order to group bacteria according to their phylogenetic origin (Lane *et al.*, 1985). Comparison of bacterial rDNA sequences has demonstrated similarities that can be categorised into cluster and sub-cluster groups. These phylogenetic trees correlated well with existing taxonomic systems, whilst also emphasising relationships that lead to the generation of new taxa.

	CFU /g wet weight	Main functional groups
Stomach	$10^7 - 10^9$	Lactobacilli
Duodenum	$10^6 - 10^8$	Lactic acid bacteria, Enterobacteria
Jejunum	$10^7 - 10^9$	Lactic acid bacteria, Strict anaerobes, Enterobacteria
Ileum	$10^8 - 10^{10}$	Strict anaerobes, lactic acid bacteria, Enterobacteria
Caecum	$10^{11} - 10^{12}$	Strict anaerobes, archaebacteria, lactic acid bacteria, Enterobacteria
Colon	$10^{10} - 10^{12}$	Strict anaerobes, Lactobacilli, Streptococci, Enterobacteria

Table 1. Total cultiviable counts of bacteria in the chyme of pigs and main functional groups.

The direct extraction of DNA from a sample, amplification of its rDNA and subsequent sequence analysis circumvents the unreliable cultivation of bacteria in a sample. Sequence comparison of rDNA amplication allows the researcher to generate phylogenetic trees and thus evaluate quality (diversity) and in part quantity of individual members of the bacterial communities in the extracted sample. The use of rDNA can also be extended to the detection of rRNA, which is the translated sequence of the rDNA blueprint. Detection of specific rRNA is advantageous for studies on bacterial metabolism, because actual metabolic activity in terms of produced ribosomes is measured.

Leser *et al.* (2002) carried out extensive 16S rDNA sequencing on the composition of ileal and hindgut bacterial communities in adult pigs in Denmark. They found that 309 from a total of 375 amplified 16s rDNA sequences (83%) were unknown, and from this it can be presumed that a majority of intestinal bacteria in the hindgut of pigs have not yet been identified. Observed functional groups of bacteria in over 4000 generated clones were similar to cultivation results, but certain species were found that were previously not regarded as indigenous or important to pigs (for instance *Streptococcus agalactolyticus*).

Much less is known about the bacterial composition in the small intestine. High flow rates restrict bacterial growth to epithelial surfaces. Although unknown mucus-associated species are being isolated (Roos *et al.*, 2000), it is conceivable that growth requirements in these habitats are even more complex than those in the hindgut.

Examples of bacterial responses to nutritional factors

Non-starch polysaccharides (NSP) and NSP hydrolysing enzymes

Arabinoxylans (pentosans) are NSP occurring in rye and especially wheat. These carbohydrates cannot be digested by host enzymes and thus tend to increase digesta viscosity in monogastric animals. However, Bartelt *et al.* (2002) measured the precaecal digestibility of arabinoxylans in piglets and reported considerable digestibility of insoluble arabinoxylans. Interestingly, the digestibility of the soluble fraction was negative (Figure 1).

Figure 1.
Digestibility of arabinose and xylose xylans in piglets (Bartelt *et al.*, 2002).

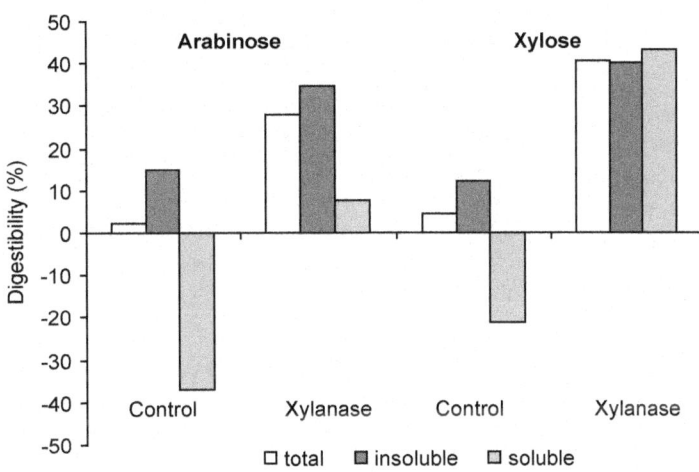

This indicates that the solubilisation of insoluble NSP occurs due to the metabolic activity of bacteria in the small intestine. When a xylanase was added to the diet, digestibility of all fractions was increased and became positive, which might be a direct effect of the exogenous enzyme, but also of a stimulated degradation by supporting a specialised group of NSP-hydrolysing bacteria.

Several studies about effect of viscosity-generating cereals and viscosity-reducing enzymes on bacterial communities in broiler chicken and piglets were carried out in our institute. From these studies a flowchart has been constructed which illustrates the expected modes of action of viscosity-generating cereals and beneficial effects of enzyme supplementation (Figure 2).

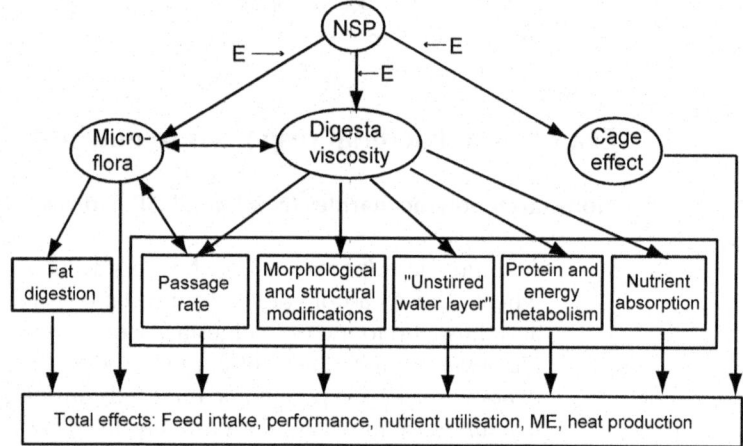

Figure 2. Flowchart for modes of action of non-starch polysaccharides and non-starch polysaccharide hydrolysing enzymes.

The main observation for poultry was a shift of NSP-degrading bacteria to more proximal parts of the intestine as a response to endogenous enzyme activity, which generates suitable substrates for some bacteria. Comparison of low viscosity (maize/ soy bean meal) vs. high viscosity diets (wheat/ rye) in broiler chickens demonstrated that bacterial beta-glucanase-degrading activities were enhanced due to a higher amount of soluble-NSP in the diet (Figure 3). Enzyme (E)-supplementation of the diet further increased glucanase-degrading activities in the small intestine, but decreased respective activities in the caeca.

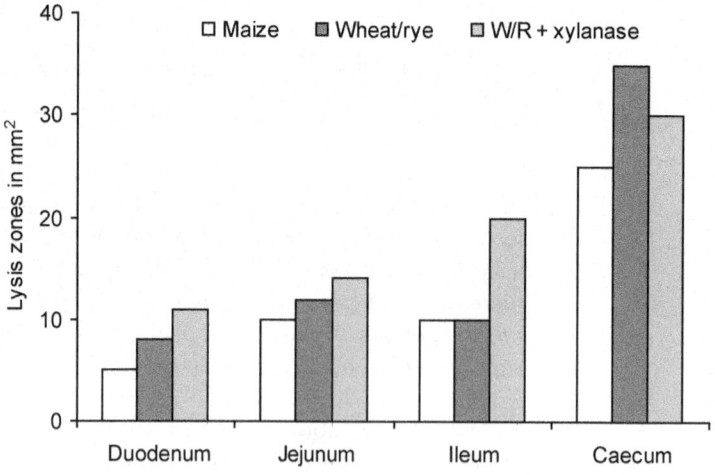

Figure 3. Beta-glucanase activity in the intestine of broiler chicken (28d).

Similar results were recorded for beta-glucan-degrading Enterococci. From our studies, Enterococci seem to be the main beta-glucan-degrading bacteria in the small intestine of poultry. A comparison of the proportion of beta-glucan-degrading Enterococci showed that up to 70% of enterococci were able to hydrolyse beta-glucans in animals fed an enzyme-supplemented wheat/ rye diet, while those receiving the non-supplemented diet only reached a maximum of 40% beta-glucan degrading Enterococci. Furthermore, by conventional techniques it was demonstrated that enzyme addition significantly reduced Enterobacteria and Gram positive cocci in the small intestine of chicken, while counts of lactic acid bacteria were increased in the same animals (Vahjen et al., 1998).

Antinutritive effects of viscosity-producing cereals in piglets are far less pronounced than in poultry. The main reason must be assigned to differences in length and volume of the intestine. The short intestinal tract of poultry requires fast flow rates in order to keep bacterial growth in check. Any delay of digesta passage in poultry will increase bacterial activity to a higher extent than in animals with longer and larger intestines. However, although viscosity related effects are small in piglets, beneficial effects on performance and precaecal amino acid digestibility have been observed in studies conducted in this laboratory. For example, the reduction of diarrhoea in enzyme-supplemented weaned piglets indicates bacterial influences within the intestine.

In a study investigating the metabolic activity of lactobacilli (detection of 16s rRNA by hybridisation) in the small intestine of piglets, we demonstrated changes in composition and subsequent activity of several lactobacilli species (Figure 4). Furthermore, the study showed increased Lactobacillus mucosae rRNA in the small intestinal lumen of control animals, which may be viewed as increased shedding of epithelial cells by the host. This supports the hypothesis that enzyme-supplemented diets decrease endogenous nitrogen loss by reduced epithelial shedding.

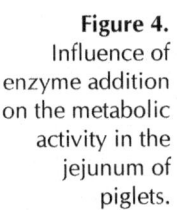

Figure 4. Influence of enzyme addition on the metabolic activity in the jejunum of piglets.

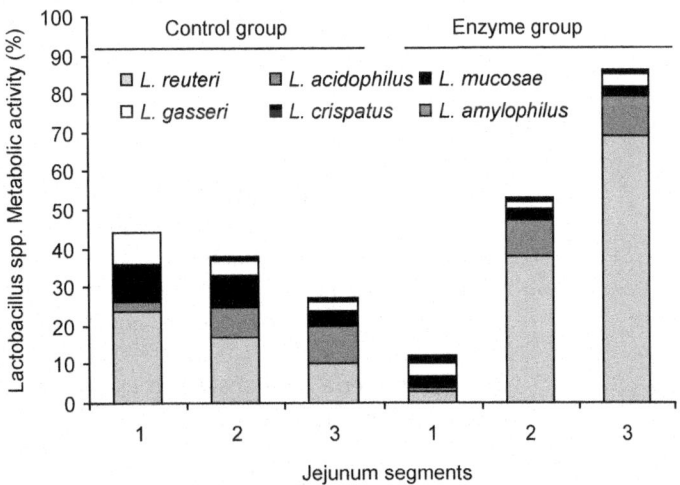

Prebiotics

Some carbohydrate fractions of the plant cell wall are thought to induce so called "prebiotic" effects in the intestine. Inulin and other mannose- or fructose-oligosaccharides are hypothesised to be fermented by only a few intestinal bacterial species, increasing the amount of beneficial bacteria like Bifidobacteria. Unfortunately, the supplemented amount of prebiotic oligosaccharides in animal diets is only a very small fraction of total carbohydrates available for bacterial fermentation. In addition, prebiotic preparations often contain significant amounts of monomer sugars that are readily consumed by intestinal bacteria. In this regard we have shown that many Enterobacteria and Streptococci are able to grow with inulin preparations as the sole energy source (Table 2).

Table 2.
Percent of
Enterobacteria
and Streptococci
isolates from
broiler chicken
capable of
growth with
a commercial
Inulin-
preparation.

Intestinal segment	Enterobacteria		Streptococci	
	number	*%*	*number*	*%*
Crop	10	30	10	80
Stomach	-	-	11	100
Jejunum	-	-	16	100
Ileum	6	100	7	100
Caecum	12	83	19	100

Nevertheless, studies investigating the influence of inulin preparations on the metabolic activity of bacterial communities in broiler chickens have indeed demonstrated an increased amount of bifidobacteria rRNA in the small intestine (Figure 5). This correlated well with increased concentrations of propionate, a typical product of bifidobacterial metabolism. Alternatively, the proposed beneficial metabolite lactate decreased, together with metabolites of strict anaerobic bacteria (butyrate, valeriate; data not shown). However, clear differences were only seen late in the fattening period, which indicates that specific traits may take a relatively long time to yield visible differences in the intestinal bacterial composition.

Probiotics

The concept of probiotics is not novel. Indeed Elie Mechnikoff originally developed it almost 100 years ago, by proposing that bacteria in fermented milk products may have the capacity to control bacterial fermentation processes in the intestine of man and may also prevent arteriosclerosis. *L. acidophilus* and other species of the genus Lactobacillus (Sanders, 2000; DiRienzo, 2000) as well as bifidobacteria are considered as probiotic bacteria with health promoting effects in humans.

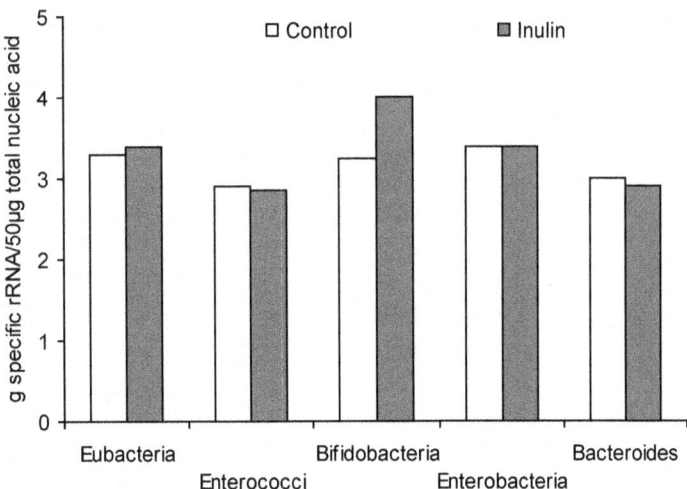

Figure 5. Metabolic activity of bacterial groups in broiler chicken.

The concept of probiotics has also been applied within the field of animal nutrition, and research in this area has heightened with the imminent ban on AGPs with the European Union. Probiotics are generally considered among other substances as candidates for alternatives to AGPs due to their beneficial effects on the gut microbiota and animal performance. The definition of probiotics in animal nutrition differs slightly from that applied in human nutrition and refers to micro-organisms which are applied as feed additives. Probiotics should lead to beneficial effects for the host animal due to an improvement of the intestinal microbial balance (according to Fuller, 1989) or of the properties of the indigenous micro-flora (according to Havernaar et al., 1992). These descriptions demonstrate that there are still relatively limited data elucidating the exact mode of action of probiotics. Most research has been performed studying the effects of lactobacilli using rodents as the model animal. However, lactobacilli are not common feed additives for farm animals.

From peformance studies carried out with pigs, it is clear that the majority of studies show trends towards positive effects. However, the significance level of $p \leq 0.05$ is only achieved in approximately 5 per cent of the experiments, which is supported by results generated in this laboratory. For example, in a trial study involving 90 control and 90 treatment (B. cereus-preparation) weaned piglets, the probiotic-treated animals gained 7% more weight during the first 6 weeks post-weaning, together with a reduced feed conversion ratio of 2.4%. However, both results were not significant (Jadamus, 2001), and show a high variation in the response of individual animals to this type of feed additive.

Diarrhoea immediately post-weaning is a principal concern for pig producers worldwide. As such, a common research area is the use of probiotics for the prophylaxis of diarrhoea, and a general suitability for this purpose has been demonstrated.

Although conventional methods provide limited results, they do allow the study of the cultivable component of the intestinal microbiota. For example, in piglets it has been demonstrated that the application of 10^8 colony forming units (CFU) of a *B. cereus* preparation per kg feed reduced counts for Lactobacilli, Bifidobacteria, Eubacteria and *E. coli* in the duodenum and jejunum, but increased respective CFU in the ileum, caecum and colon (Gedek *et al.*, 1993). A significant reduction of *E. coli* CFU in the small intestine of piglets was also noted in a study using an *E. faecium* preparation (Männer and Spieler, 1997). However, in the same study there was a strong trend towards increased Lactobacilli, whilst Enterococci counts increased significantly. Furthermore, Jadamus *et al.* (2000) reported a reduction in the colonisation of mucosa-associated enterobacteria with the use of a probiotic *B. cereus* preparation. The use of an *in vitro* method (bacterial growth capacities of mucosal samples incubated in liquid selective media) also shows that *B. cereus* reduces the development of mucosa-associated Enterobacteria in suckling piglets. However, the effect was demised as piglets aged and growth capacities changed after weaning (Jadamus *et al.*, 2000).

In an attempt to more closely monitor the metabolic activity of indigenous intestinal bacteria in turkey poults, we have used rRNA targeted probes specific for Lactobacilli, Enterococci and Enterobacteria in order to investigate probiotic modifications for these groups of bacteria (Vahjen *et al.*, 2002). The results indicate that the probiotic *E. faecium* strain enhanced metabolic activity of Lactobacilli (Figure 6) and increased lactate concentration. Differences in colony counts of lactic acid bacteria (MRS medium) were only apparent on the 28th day of life (data not shown).

Conversely, due to the high inclusion rate of the probiotic *E. faecium* strain, enterococci counts were always higher in the treatment group up to a saturation threshold of about 10^5/g wet weight. However, comparisons between control- and treatment-groups using probe hybridisations showed similar activity on the 7th day of life with higher activity only observed later on the 28th and 35th day of life, corresponding to colony count peak levels. These comparative results demonstrate that a high discriminatory power is required to study probiotic effects on indigenous bacteria. Quantitative techniques that target specific bacterial rRNA content, possibly combined with the measurement of specific enzyme activities and

Figure 6.
Effect of a
probiotic
E. faecium
preparation on the
16S RNA-content
of Lactobacillus
spp. in the small
intestine of turkeys.

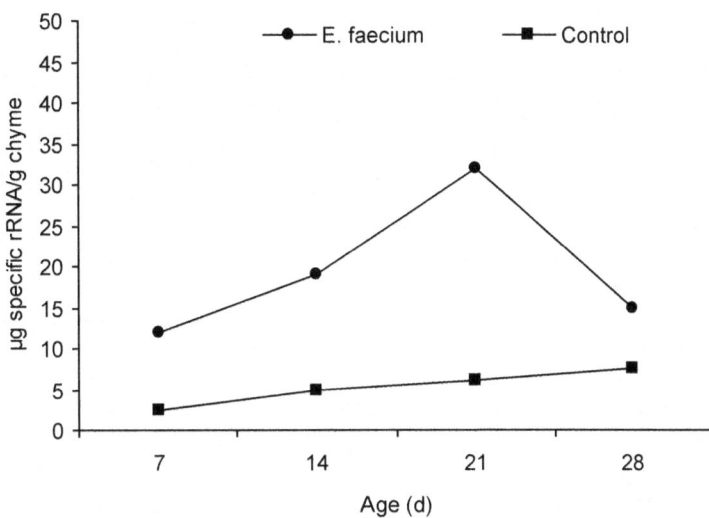

products are preferable. Indirect analysis via cultivation or amplification of DNA can only yield cell number or potential activity in terms of amplified DNA copies.

Extensive studies on bacterial composition and activity concerning the effects of probiotics in pigs are performed at this institute involving an interdisciplinary research group. From current results, one major probiotic effect is created by modification of bacterial communities of nursing sows receiving the probiotic-supplemented diet. Using the denaturing gradient gel electrophoresis (DGGE) and construction of similarity indices, we observed that banding patterns from probiotic-fed piglets (suckling) clustered in similar groups, while animals fed the unsupplemented diet exhibited more diverse clusters (Figure 7). These results indicate that, analogous to prebiotics, probiotics may need time and daily supplementation to exert any beneficial effects. These experiments are currently in their infancy, thus data are not yet available for in-depth discussion. However, various modifications of the microbial community, structure and function of intestinal tissues and the response of the immune system are indicated.

Summary

The whole gastrointestinal tract of monogastric animals is colonised by micro-organisms with highly variable metabolic potentials. Their metabolic activity and cell numbers are most pronounced in the hindgut. However significant bacterial nutrient conversion occurs in the small intestine, which is also the major site for host immune response and thus critical to the health status of the animal.

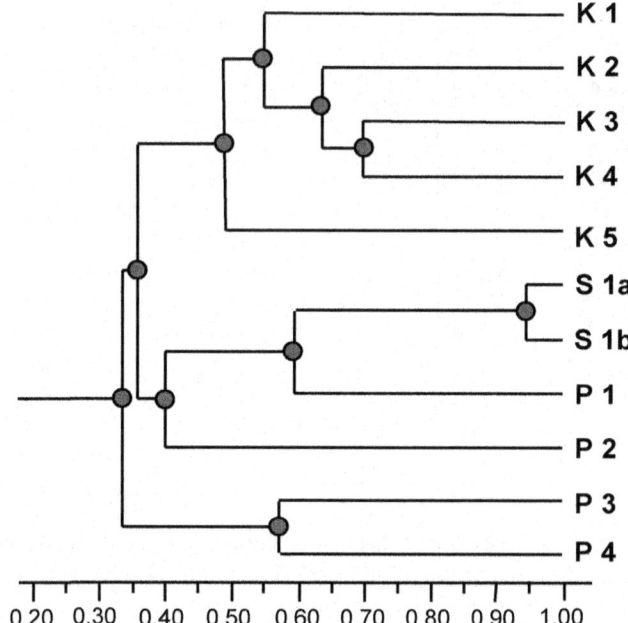

Actual knowledge concerning the biodiversity of intestinal microbiota is somewhat limited due to various methodological problems. In addition to cultural techniques, new techniques based on detection of bacterial ribosomal nucleic acids are available and will support our gain of knowledge within this field.

This chapter provides examples covering the interaction of nutritional factors with intestinal bacteria. It has been shown that elevated NSP concentrations in feed stimulate a specific functional group of bacteria which produce NSP-hydrolysing enzymes. Evidence in chickens suggests that the addition of a xylanase to a diet rich in arabinoxylans induces a shift of this specific microbial population towards proximal segments of the intestine. Furthermore, it was shown that studies on the response of bacteria to nutritional factors require techniques that are sensitive on the species level. Additionally, feed additives aimed to beneficially modify the intestinal microflora were studied. Probiotic bacteria do modify intestinal microbial populations, however, at present interpretation of underlying probiotic mechanisms including interactions with the epithelial tissue or the immune system are still of a hypothetical character.

References

Bartelt, J., Jadamus, A., Wiese, F., Swiech, E., Buraczewska, L., and Simon, O. (2002) Apparent precaecal digestibility of nutrients and level of endogenous nitrogen in digesta of the small intestine of growing pigs as affected by various digesta viscosities. *Archives of Animal Nutrition* **56**: 93-107.

DiRienzo, D.B. (2000) Symposium: Probiotic bacteria: Implications for human health. *Journal of Nutrition* **130**: 382S-383S.

Fuller, R. (1989) Probiotics in man and animals. *Journal of Applied Bacteriology* **66**: 365-378.

Havernaar, R., Ten Brink, B., and Huis in't Veld, J.H.J. (1992) Selection of strains for probiotic use. In: *Probiotics. The scientific basis*. Edited by Fuller R. pp. 209-224. Chapman and Hall, London.

Jadamus, A., Vahjen, W., and Simon, O. (2000) Influence of the probiotic bacterial strain, *Bacillus cereus* var. toyoi, on the development of selected microbial groups adhering to intestinal mucosal tissues of piglets. *Journal of Animal and Feed Science* **9**: 347-362.

Jadamus, A. (2001) Untersuchungen zur Wirksamkeit und Wirkungsweise des sporenbildenden *Bacillus cereus* var. toyoi im Verdauungstrakt von Broilern und Ferkel, Doctoral Thesis at the Free University, Berlin.

Gedek, B., Kirchgessner, M., Wiehler, S., Bott, A., Eidelsburger, U., and Roth, F.X. (1993) Zur nutritiven Wirksamkeit von *Bacillus cereus* als Probiotikum in der Ferkelaufzucht. 2. Mitteilung – Einfluss auf Keimzahlen, Zusammensetzung und Resistenzeigenschaften der gastrointestinalen und faecalen Mikroflora. *Archives of Animal Nutrition* **44**: 215-226

Lane, D. J., Pace, B., Olsen, G. J., Stahl, D. A., Sogin, M. L., and Pace, N. R. (1985) Rapid determination of 16S ribosomal RNA Sequences for phylogenetic analysis. *Proceedings of the National Acadademy of Science* USA **82**: 6955-6959.

Meyerholz, D. K, Stabel, T. J., and Cheville, N. F. (2002) Segmented filamentous bacteria interact with intraepithelial mononuclear cells. *Infection and Immunity* **70**(6):3277-3280.

Roos, S., Karner, F., Axelsson, L., and Jonsson, H. (2000) *Lactobacillus mucosae* sp. nov., a new species with *in vitro* mucus-binding activity isolated from pig intestine. *International Journal of Systems of Evolutionary Microbiology* **50**: 251-258.

Sanders, M.E. (2000) Consideration for use of probiotic bacteria to modulate human health. Symposium: Probiotic bacteria: Implications for human health. *Journal of Nutrition* **130**: 384S-390S.

Vahjen, W., Glaeser, K., and Simon, O. (1998) Influence of xylanase supplemented feed on the development of selected bacterial groups in the intestinal tract of broiler chicks. *Journal of Agricultural Science* **130**: 489-500.

Vahjen, W., Jadamus, A., and Simon, O. (2002) Influence of a probiotic *Enterococcus faecium* strain on selected bacterial groups in the small intestine of growing turkey poults. *Archives of Animal Nutrition* **56**: 419-429.

Commensal bacteria and intestinal development: Studies using gnotobiotic pigs

Andrew Van Kessel, T.W. Shirkey, R.H. Siggers, M.D. Drew, B. Laarveld
Department of Animal and Poultry Science, University of Saskatchewan, Saskatoon, SK, S7N 5A8, Canada

Introduction

Soon after birth the intestine of the pig is colonized by coliform bacteria followed rapidly by predominantly anaerobic bacteria and becoming more complex with age (Swords *et al.*,1993). Estimates suggest 500 or more bacterial species colonize the adult intestine reaching 10^{11} cfu/g intestinal contents and totalling 10-fold more cells than the number of cells in the pig's body. Furthermore, the aggregate genome of these bacteria represent 2-4 million genes in contrast to only 30 to 40 000 genes present in the host genome (Hooper and Gordon, 2001). Comparisons of conventional and gnotobiotic (germ-free or having a defined microbiota) animals have indicated a marked host response to bacterial colonization of the intestine as evidenced by obvious contrasts in intestinal morphology, immunity and digestive function (Coates *et al.*,1963; Pabst *et al.*,1988; Wostmann, 1996).

Recently, Hooper *et al.* (2001) used genome-wide expression profiling in gnotobiotic rodents to confirm a marked effect of the commensal bacteria and uncovered a tremendous array of intestinal genes regulated by bacterial colonization, including genes involved in nutrient uptake and metabolism (e.g. sodium glucose contransporter (SGLT-1), co-lipase) and mucosal barrier function (e.g. sprr2a, decay accelerating factor). Most interestingly, expression profiling in gnotobiotic animal studies, and the results of *in vitro* studies using bacterial co-culture with intestinal epithelial cell lines indicate that host gene expression responses are specific for different bacteria. As a result, the composition of the commensal bacteria colonizing the neonatal intestine may have significant consequences relative to intestinal development, immunity and the digestion and absorption of nutrients. The following paper reviews bacteria-host interrelationships with particular reference to the impact of the intestinal commensal bacteria on the development and function of the intestine. We will highlight the breadth of the host responses

47

observed in relation to intestinal microbiota as well as evidence indicating that the composition of the commensal bacteria can have significant developmental and function consequences in the intestine.

Production performance

Increased performance parameters have been reported in gnotobiotic (bacteria or 'germ'-free) versus conventional chickens (Coates *et al.*,1963; Yokota and Coates, 1982; Muramatsu *et al.*, 1988; Furuse *et al.*, 1991; Furuse and Yokota, 1994). However, there is very little information published on growth rate in gnotobiotic pigs. Shurson *et al.* (1990) investigated the physiological relationship between copper and microbiological environment and reported that gnotobiotic pigs tended to have increased average daily gain (ADG) associated primarily with increased average daily feed intake (ADFI) rather than improved feed efficiency. Using a small number of pigs we observed increased growth rate in pigs colonized by 3 species of bacteria compared with pigs colonized by a complex microbiota and reared to 26 days of age (Shirkey *et al.*, 2003). Due to the small number of animals that can typically be reared under germ-free conditions and the effect of sterilization procedures on the nutrient content of diets, accurate assessment of performance traits is difficult in the pig.

Intestinal morphology

A marked adaptive response of the gut to colonization by bacteria is evident by comparison of small intestinal morphology and function between gnotobiotic- and conventionally- reared animals. Morphologic changes in gnotobiotic animals include a reduction in intestinal mass per unit length, intestinal thickness and length (Wostmann, 1996). Studies conducted in this laboratory have revealed similar changes in intestinal morphology in the gnotobiotic pig including a significant increase in small intestinal length at 13 days of age (unpublished). Much of the reduction in intestinal mass and thickness in gnotobiotic animals is related to a markedly reduced cellularity of the *lamina propria*, which in conventional animals is populated by lymphoid, mesenchymal, nerve and vascular cells (Gaskins, 1997). Interestingly, in our experiments a marked increase in villus height, observed in the distal small intestine of germ-free and gnotobiotic pigs (see below), more than compensated for the loss of mass associated with reduced lamina propria cellularity.

The mucosal surface of the intestine is characterized by finger-like projections called villi and mucosal invaginations called the crypts of

Lieberkühn. In gnotobiotic animals, villi are long, thin and regularly shaped, while crypts are relatively short resulting in an increased villus:crypt ratio as compared to conventional animals (Kentworthy, 1970; Heneghan, 1984; Wostmann, 1996). Interestingly, we noticed that intestinal epithelial cells lining the villi in the distal small intestine of gnotobiotic and mono-associated pigs had an extremely vacuolated appearance, particularly at the villus tips. These "foamy" villi were first described by Kentworthy (1970) which under the electron microscope showed numerous smooth surfaced vesicles that contained a 'mottled amorphous material of moderate to slight electron density'. Jensen et al. (2001) observed these vacuoles in 2-d-old colostrum-deprived conventional pigs and suggested these vacuoles were the result of incomplete macromolecular absorption when passive antibody is supplied without colostrum.

Figure 1 illustrates villus height:crypt depth ratio along the length of the small intestine in 13-day old gnotobiotic (GF) pigs, ex-gnotobiotic pigs conventionalized by inoculation with feces (CV), and ex-gnotobiotic pigs mono-associated with *Lactobacillus fermentum* (LF) or a non-pathogenic *Escherichia coli* (EC) (Shirkey et al., 2003). Villus height was up to 3 times greater in gnotobiotic versus conventionalized pigs in the distal small intestine where bacterial colonization is typically highest in conventional pigs. Villus height and crypt depth were not significantly different between gnotobiotic and *L. fermentum* groups, however, *E. coli* mono-association appeared to reduce villus height and increase crypt depth.

Figure 1. Villus characteristics along the small intestine (pyloric sphincter = 0; ileo cecal junction = 100) in 13-day-old mono-associated and conventionalized isolator-reared pigs.

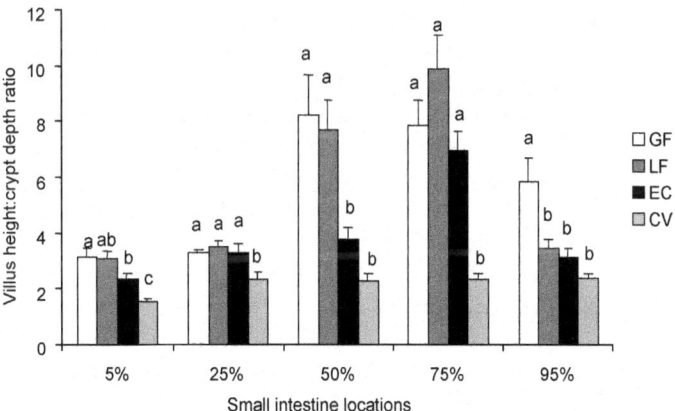

Within intestinal section, bars with different letters are significantly (P<0.05) different

Intestinal epithelial cells lining the intestinal mucosal surface undergo a process of continual renewal. Four lineages of epithelial cells develop from stem cells located in the crypts including absorptive enterocytes (>80% of all epithelial cells), mucus secreting goblet cells, entero-endocrine cells and Paneth cells (Falk *et al.*, 1998). With the exception of Paneth cells that remain in the crypts, newly generated epithelial cells mature as they migrate towards the villus tip where they are exfoliated (Falk *et al.*, 1998). In the absence of bacteria, the transit time of an epithelial cell from crypt to villus tip may be increased by a factor of 2 (Wostmann, 1996). In agreement with our findings regarding villus:crypt ratio in the pig (Figure 1), differences in the magnitude of epithelial cell renewal between gnotobiotic and conventional chickens were reported greatest in distal areas of the gut where microbial populations are highest (Rolls *et al.*, 1978). Also in agreement with our observations in the pig, monoassociation of mice with a strain of a *Lactobacillus* sp. produced no noticeable effect on intestinal morphology and renewal rate compared with conventional mice (Savage *et al.*, 1981). In contrast, Kentworthy and Allen, (1966) observed that pigs monoassociated with either *E. coli* or *Staphylococcus albus* exhibited an increase in the mitotic index, deeper crypts and shorter villi.

Recently, glucagon-like peptide 2 (GLP-2), one of several cleavage products of proglucagon, has been identified as a primary regulator of intestinal epithelial cell renewal (Burrin *et al.*, 2001). To determine the effect of commensal bacteria on proglucagon expression, we measured the abundance of porcine proglucagon mRNA in intestine of the gnotobiotic pigs described in Figure 1 (Siggers *et al.*, 2003). In the distal small intestine, proglucagon transcript abundance was not different between germ-free and conventionalized pigs. However, *L. fermentum* monoassociation tended to increase transcript abundance about 2 fold whereas *E. coli* monoassociation tended to decrease transcript abundance versus germ-free pigs. While the association between proglucagon transcript abundance and intestinal mucosal morphology is not clear, it is clear that the composition of the commensal intestinal bacteria can markedly affect host gene expression responses.

Mucus secretion

The gastrointestinal epithelium is covered by a layer of mucus, which forms a boundary between the lumen contents and the mucosa (Forstner and Forstner, 1994). Mucus offers several ecological benefits to the intestinal bacteria. Mucin oligosaccharides provide a source of carbohydrates and peptides for bacterial proliferation and bacteria that are able to colonize mucus can avoid expulsion during gastric emptying and intestinal peristalsis (Deplancke and Gaskins, 2001). Alternatively, as a host defence strategy, mucus may provide competitive attachment sites for pathogens, preventing direct attachment of pathogens to the epithelial cell surface. Thus, as proposed in a recent review of mucus secretion by Deplancke and Gaskins, (2001), it would be considered advantageous for commensal and pathogenic bacteria to chemically regulate mucus synthesis and secretion.

Mucus is secreted from specialized epithelial cells called goblet cells. The effect of commensal intestinal microbiota on goblet cell number appears to depend on location within the intestine. Goblet cells are increased in number in the small intestine of gnotobiotic rodents, dogs and pigs (Kandori et al., 1996; Wostmann, 1996; unpublished). However, goblets cells are fewer in number and smaller in size in the caecum and colon of gnotobiotic rodents relative to conventionally-raised rodents (Ishikawa et al., 1989; Sharma and Scumacher, 1995). The mucus layer in the colon and caecum of conventional rodents has also been reported to be up to twice as thick compared to gnotobiotic rodents (Kandori et al., 1996; Meslin et al., 1999) suggesting increased mucus secretion.

Bacterial colonization of the intestine may also affect mucus composition. Comparison of the number of goblet cells staining for neutral mucins, acid mucins or sulfomucins and the staining density among gnotobiotic rats and rats harbouring conventional microbiota or human microbiota indicated marked effects of the intestinal microbiota (Sharma and Scumacher, 1995). A remarkable regulation of mucin composition was first reported by Bry et al. (1996) using gnotobiotic mice reconstituted with Bacteroides thetaiotaomicron. This bacterium was capable of inducing intestinal epithelial cell expression of α1,2-fucosyltransferase resulting in fucosylation of glycoconjugates. Strikingly, an isogenic strain of B. thetaiotaomicron, incapable of fucose catabolism, was not able to induce α1,2-fucosyltransferase expression. The ability to activate fucosylytransferase mRNA was dependent on the ability to sense L-fucose in the environment and regulate expression of an operon controlling fucose metabolism and an uncharacterized locus responsible for fucosylytransferase induction in epithelial cells (Hooper et al., 1999).

The gel-forming properties of mucus are attributed largely to glycoproteins, cell mucins for which 9 epithelial mucin (MUC) genes have been identified in humans (Deplancke and Gaskins, 2001). There is good evidence that mucin gene expression is differentially regulated by the intestinal bacteria. For example, co-incubation of an entero-pathogenic E. coli strain with HT-29 cells did not affect MUC 2 or MUC 3 expression, however, Lactobacillus plantarum 299v and L. rhamnosus GG caused an increase in expression of these genes (Mack *et al.*, 1999). The authors proposed that the ability of these probiotic strains to regulate mucin production might be related to their ability to prevent *E. coli* adherence to HT-29 cells. Bacteria may also inhibit mucin production within the intestine. Byrd *et al.* (2000) established that mucin synthesis was inhibited more than 80% when KATO III cells were incubated for a prolonged period with *Helicobacter pylori*.

Bacterial regulation of mucin synthesis and secretion may also occur indirectly through host-derived cytokines. Enss *et al.* (2000) measured MUC expression levels in the intestinal cancer cell line LS180 that were exposed to a variety of pro-inflammatory cytokines. Incubation with IL-1 stimulated expression of MUC 2 and MUC 5AC, whereas IL-6 up-regulated an early response of MUC 2, MUC 5B and MUC 6. TNF-α induced expression of MUC 2 and MUC 5B for 3 hours, and had no effect on the expression of MUC 5AC and MUC 6. Interestingly, the pro-inflammatory cytokines stimulated the release of less glycosylated mucins, which may be due to accelerated passage of the mucin molecule through the Golgi complex.

Nutrient digestion and metabolism

Little information is available on the effects of the commensal microbiota on stomach function although Coring *et al.* (1981) report HCl secretion is increased 2.7 fold in gnotobiotic rats. The secretion of pancreatic proteolytic enzymes including trypsinogen, chymotrypsinogen, amylase, lipase, carboxypeptidases A and B and elastase, do not appear to be influenced by commensal bacteria (Bruckner and Szabó, 1984). However, bacteria may indirectly alter host enzyme activity through luminal pH changes and gradual microbial inactivation (Bruckner and Szabó, 1984). In the gnotobiotic animal, for example, digestive enzyme activity in intestinal contents does not decrease along the length of the intestine as observed in conventional animals (Bruckner and Szabó, 1984). Increased specific activity of brush border disaccharidases and peptidases has been observed in gnotobiotic rodents, pigs and chickens associated with a reduced rate of epithelial cell replacement and increased the number of mature epithelial cells (Bruckner and Szabó, 1984; Wostmann, 1996).

Immunity and cytokine expression

The gastrointestinal tract represents an enormous surface area that on the one hand must be permeable to an array of nutrients while on the other, an efficient barrier against entrance of pathogens. Protection of the intestinal surface includes a range of physical and innate defence mechanisms as well as an elaborate active mucosal defence mechanism. Much of the study of the intestinal mucosal immune defence has focused on active immunity characterized by the uptake of antigen across specialized M cells, the activation of specific T- and B-cells in specialized lymphoid follicles called Peyer's patches, and the trafficking of effectors cells into the *lamina propria*. These effectors cells mount protective responses against specific pathogens including cellular and humoral effector mechanisms. Intriguingly, in the vast majority of cases (via mechanisms that are poorly understood), the mucosal immune system is able to mount strong protective responses against invasive organisms while remaining tolerant of food antigens and indeed, non invasive commensal organisms.

In gnotobiotic animals, development of gut-associated lymphoid tissue is markedly slowed, although not arrested. Jejunal and ileal Peyer's patches are reduced in size by about 50% in gnotobiotic versus conventional pigs (Pabst *et al.*, 1988). The reduction in mucosal immune response and the associated infiltration of effector immune cells into the *lamina propria* accounts largely for the decrease in intestine thickness observed in gnotobiotic animals (Furse and Okumura, 1994). In the pig, the increase in number of intraepithelial lymphocytes (IEL), which migrate into the epithelial layer from the *lamina propria*, occurs with maturation in the conventionally reared pig, but is absent in gnotobiotic pigs (Rothkotter *et al.*, 1999).

Additionally, we have observed small but easily distinguishable Peyer's patches, markedly reduced cellularity of the *lamina propria* and a 2-3 fold decrease in the number of IEL in the intestinal epithelium of 13-day-old gnotobiotic pigs. Interestingly, although cellularity of the *lamina propria* was marginally increased, the number of IEL in pigs monoassociated with *L. fermentum* or a non-pathogenic *E. coli* was not different from gnotobiotic pigs (Shirkey, 2003) indicating a remarkable ability of the immune system to respond according to the level of bacterial invasiveness. In the mouse, immunological responses to commensal bacteria are transient and gradually wane (Shroff *et al.*, 1995), however, acute responses range from weak to moderate, to severe (McCracken and Gaskins, 1999) and there appears to be no current categorization of bacteria which would predict the degree of response in gnotobiotic animals (e.g. some Gram-negative strains may be weakly or strongly immunogenic in gnotobiotic animals).

Recently, it has been recognized that intestinal epithelial cells are immuno-competent cells and are likely to be important participants in intestinal immune networks. Intestinal epithelial cells express

MHC class II antigens in response to IFNγ and may present antigen to lymphocytes in the *lamina propria* (Hecht and Savkovic, 1997). Epithelial cells also express a variety of cytokines common to antigen presenting cell lineages including the pro-inflammatory cytokines IL-1α, IL-1ß, TNFα, IL-6 and IL-8 and the anti-inflammatory cytokines TGF-ß, and IL-10 (Hecht and Savkovic, 1997; Autschbach *et al.*,1998).

The ability of intestinal epithelial cells to respond differentially to bacteria has been demonstrated in studies employing cultured epithelial cell lines. Delneste *et al.* (1998) examined the immunological effects of two lactobacillus (LAB) strains and a non-pathogenic *E. coli* on a human colonic epithelial cell line (HT-29 cells). Expression of pro-inflammatory cytokines (TNFα, IL-8, GM-CSF, MCP-I) was increased by exposure of HT-29 to *E. coli*, but LAB generally did not alter the cytokine profile from baseline. Addition of IFNγ to the media increased the inflammatory cytokine response to *E. coli* but not LAB. Intestinal epithelial cells require IFNγ for induction of MHC class II expression (Hecht and Savkovic, 1997). Interestingly, both *E. coli* and LAB augmented the MHC class II response to IFNγ. McCracken *et al.* (2002) determined that IL-8 mRNA expression was not detectable by Northern blot analysis in HT-29 colonic cells that were cultured with *Lactobacillus plantarum* 299v. However, HT-29 cells that were co-cultured with TNF-a and *L. plantarum* 299v resulted in significant increase in IL-8 expression.

Pro-inflammatory cytokines associated with the acute phase response (IL-I, TNFα and IL-6) have been shown to suppress feed intake, increase degradation of muscle protein, increase lipolysis in adipocytes (Klasing and Johnstone, 1991; Spurlock, 1997) and directly modulate intestinal nutrient transport by IEC (Hardin *et al.*, 2000). In an attempt to understand whether the composition of the commensal intestinal microbiota could directly affect host performance through modulation of intestinal cytokine expression, we examined IL-1 and IL-6 expression in whole intestinal sections obtained from gnotobiotic pigs, pigs inoculated with adult pig feces (conventionalized) and pigs mono-associated with *L. fermentum* or non-pathogenic *E. coli* (Shirkey *et al.*, 2003). Interestingly, in the distal small intestine, the highest level of IL-1 expression was observed in pigs mono-associated with *E. coli*. IL-1 expression was not different between the *L. fermentum* and gnotobiotic pigs and were about 20-40% of levels observed in conventionalized pigs (Figure 2). IL-6 expression followed a similar pattern as IL-1.

These results indicate that host intestine can alter cytokine production due to different signals produced by commensal bacterial populations, which may be important in regulating the state of inflammatory activation within the intestine. The molecular mechanisms involved in bacterial-induced changes in epithelial cytokine gene expression remain unknown. Understanding the epithelial cell's ability to differentiate between pathogenic and non-pathogenic adherent bacteria may provide information valuable for developing strategies to prevent colonization by pathogenic species (Gaskins, 1997). In addition, cytokine expression as affected by the composition of the commensal intestinal microbiota could have implications for the development and function of the intestine as well as animal performance.

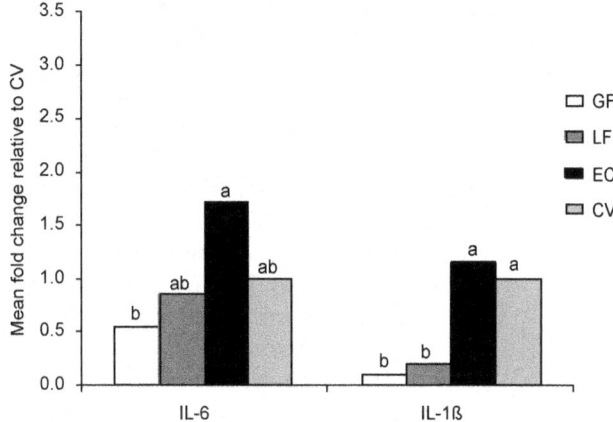

Figure 2. Interleukin(IL)-6 and IL-1ß mRNA abundance in distal small intestine of monoassociated and conventionalized isolator-reared pigs at 13 days of age.

Conclusion

The intestine is colonized by a complex community of micro-organisms 10-fold greater in number than somatic cells in the body. The intestinal microbiota forms an important barrier against pathogens and plays key roles in nutrient digestion and development of immunity. There is now clear evidence that the intestinal microbiota impact numerous gene expression pathways affecting a wide range of host functions. Elucidation of these pathways and their differential regulation by diverse commensal bacteria will lead to new approaches to modulate intestinal development, immunity and the digestion and absorption of nutrients.

References

Autschbach, F., Braunstein, J., Helmke, B., Zuna, I., Schurmann, G., Niemir, Z.I., Wallich, R., Otto, H.F., and Meuer, S.C. (1998) In situ expression of interleukin-10 in non-inflamed human gut and in inflammatory bowel disease. *American Journal of Pathology* **153**: 121-130.

Brucker, G., and Szabó, J. (198)4. Nutrient absorption in gnotobiotic animals. *Advanced Nutrition. Research* **6**: 271-332.

Bry, L., Falk, P.G., Midtvedt, T., and Gordon, J.I. (1996) A model of host-microbial interactions in an open mammalian ecosystem. *Science* **273**: 1380-1383.

Burrin, D. G., Petersen, Y., Stoll, B., and Sangild, P. (2001) Glucagon-like peptide 2: A nutrient-responsive gut growth factor. *Journal of Nutrition* **131**: 709-712.

Byrd, J.C., Yunker, C.K., Xu, Q.S., Sternberg, L.R., and Bresalier, R.S. (2000) Inhibition of gastric mucin synthesis by *Helicobacter pylori*. *Gasteroenterology* **118**: 1072-1079.

Coates, M.E., Fuller, R., Harrison, G.F., Lev, M., and Suffolk, S.F. (1963) A comparison of the growth of chicks in the Gustafsson germ-free apparatus and in a conventional environment, with and without dietary supplements of penicillin. *British Journal of Nutrition* **17**: 141-151.

Corring, T., Juste, C., and Simoes-Nunes, C. (1981) Digestive enzymes in the germ-free animal. *Reproduction and Nutrition Development* **21**: 355-370.

Delneste, Y., Donnet-Hughes, A., and Schiffrin, E.J. (1998) Functional foods: Mechanisms of action on immunocompetent cells. *Nutrition Reviews* **56**: S93-S98.

Deplancke, B., and Gaskins, H.R. (2001) Microbial modulation of innate defense: goblet cells and the intestinal mucus layer. *American Journal of Clinical Nutrition* **73**: 1131S-1141S.

Enss, M.L., Cornberg, M., Wagner, S., Gebert, A., Henrichs, M., Eisenblatter, R., Beil, W., Kownatzki, R., and Hedrich, H.J. (2000) Proinflammatory cytokines trigger MUC gene expression and mucin release in the intestinal cancer cell line LS180. *Inflammation Research* **49**: 162-69.

Falk, P.G., Hooper, L.V., Midtvedt, T., and Gordon, J.I. (1998) Creating and maintaining the gastrointestinal ecosystem: what we know and need to know from gnotobiology. *Microbiology and Molecular Biology Reviews* **62**: 1157-1170.

Forstner, J.F., and Forstner, G.G. (1994) Gastrointestinal mucus. In: *Physiology of the Gastrointestinal Tract*. Edited by Johnson, L.R. pp. 1255-1283. Raven Press, New York,

Furse, M., and Okumura, J. (1994) Nutritional and physiological characteristics in germ-free chickens. *Comparative Biochemistry and Physiology* **109A**: 547-556.

Furuse, M., Yang, S.I., Niwa, N., Choi, Y.H., Okumura, J. (1991) Energy utilization in germ-free and conventional chicks fed diets containing sorbose. *British Poultry Science* **32**: 383-390.

Gaskins, H.R. (1997) Immunological aspects of host/microbiota interactions at the intestinal epithelium. In: *Gastrointestinal Microbiology*: Vol 2. Gastrointestinal Microbiology and Host Interactions. Edited by Mackie, R.I., White, B.A., Isaacson, R.E. pp. 537-587. Chapman and Hall, New York.

Hardin, J., Kroeker, K., Chung, B. and Gall, D.G. (2000) Effect of proinflammatory interleukins on jejunal nutrient transport.

Gut **47**: 184-191.

Hecht, G. and Savkovic, S.D. (1997) Review article: Effector role of epithelia in inflammation-interaction with bacteria. *Alimentary Pharmacology Therapy* **11**(Suppl 3): 64-68.

Heneghan, J.B. (1984) Physiology of the alimentary tract. In: *The germ-free animal in biomedical research*. Edited by Coates, M.E. and Gustafsson B.E. pp. 285-289. Laboratory Animals Ltd., London.

Hooper, L.V., Xu, J., Falk, P.G., Midtvedt, T. and Gordon, J.I. (1999) A molecular sensor that allows a gut commensal to control its nutrient foundation in a competitive ecosystem. *Proceedings of the National Academy of Science* **96**: 9833-9838.

Hooper, L.V., Wong, M.H., Thelin, A., Hansson, L., Falk, P.G., and Gordon, J.I. (2001) Molecular analysis of commensal host-microbial relationships in the intestine. *Science* **291**: 881-884.

Hooper, L.V. and Gordon, J.I. (2001) Commensal host bacterial relationships in the gut. *Science* **292**: 1115-1118.

Ishikawa, K., Satoh, Y., Oomori, Y., Yamano, M., Matsuda, M. and Ono, K. (1989) Influence of conventionalization on cecal wall structure of germ-free Wistar rats: Quantitative light and qualitative electron microscopic observations. *Anatomy and Embryology* (Berl.) **180**: 191-198.

Jensen, A.R., Elnif, J., Burrin, D.G. and Sangild, P.T. (2001) Development of intestinal immunoglobulin absorption and enzyme activities in neonatal pigs is diet dependent. *Journal of Nutrition* **131**: 3259-3265.

Kandori, H., Hirayama, K., Takeda, M., and Doi, K. (1996) Histochemical, lectin-histochemical and morphometrical characteristics of intestinal goblet cells of germfree and conventional mice. *Experimental Animals* **45**: 155-160.

Kentworthy, R. (1970) Effect of Escherichia coli on germ-free and gnotobiotic pigs. I. Light and electron microscopy of the small intestine. *Journal of Comparative Pathology* **80**: 53-63.

Kentworthy, R., and Allen, W.D. (1966) Influence of diet and bacteria on small intestinal morphology, with special reference to early weaning and *Escherichia coli*. *Journal of Comparative Pathology* **76**: 291-298.

Klasing, K.C., and Johnstone, B.J. (1991) Monokines in growth and development. *Poultry Science* **70**: 1781-1789.

Mack, D.R., Michail, S., Wei, S., McDougall, L., and Hollingsworth, M.A. (1999) Probiotics inhibit Enteropathogenic *E. coli* adherence in vitro by inducing intestinal mucin gene expression. *American Journal of Gastro-intestinal Physiolology and Liver Physiology* **276**: G941-G950.

McCracken, V.J., Chun, T., Baldeon, M.E., Ahrne, S., Molin, G., Mackie, R.I., and Gaskins, H.R. (2002) TNF-alpha sensitizes HT-29 colonic epithelial cells to intestinal lactobacilli.

Experimental Biology and Medicine **227**: 665-670.

McCracken, V.J., and Gaskins, H.R. (1999) Probiotics and the immune system. In: *Probiotics: a critical review* Edited by G.W. Tannock. pp. 85-111. Horizon Scientific Press, Norfolk, UK.

Meslin, J.C., Fontaine, N. and Andrieux, C. (1999) Variation of mucin distribution in the rat intestine, cecum and colon: Effect of bacterial flora. *Comparative Biochemistry and Physiology* **123**: 235-239.

Muramatsu, T., Takasu, O., Furuse, M., and Okumura, J. (1988) Effect of diet type on enhanced intestinal protein synthesis by the gut microflora in the chick. *Journal of Nutrition* **118**: 1068-1074.

Pabst, R., Geist, M., Rothkotter, H.J. and Fritz, F.J. (1988) Postnatal development and lymphocyte production of jejunal and ileal Peyer's patches in normal and gnotobiotic pigs. *Immunology* **64**: 539-544.

Rothkotter, H.J., Mollhoff, S. and Pabst, R. (1999) The influence of age and breeding conditions on the number and proliferation of intraepithelial lymphocytes in pigs. *Scandinavian Journal of Immunology* **50**: 31-38.

Savage, D.C., Siegel, J.E., Snellen, J.E., and Whitt, D.D. (1981) Transit time of epithelial cells in the small intestines of germfree mice and ex-germfree mice associated with indigenous microorganisms. *Applied Environmental Microbiology* **42**: 996-1001.

Shirkey, T. W. (2003) Commensal bacteria differentially affect intestinal morphology and expression of pro-inflammatory cytokines in the pig. M.Sc. Thesis, University of Saskatchewan, Saskatchewan.

Shirkey, T.W., Goldade, B.G., Siggers, R.H., Drew, M.D., Laarveld, B. and Van Kessel, A.G. (2003) Effect of commensal bacteria on intestinal morphology and expression of pro-inflammatory cytokine genes in the gnotobiotic pig. *Proceedings of the 9ᵗʰ International Symposium on the Digestive Physiology of Pigs.* **2**: 290-292

Shurson, G.C., Ku, P.K., Waxler, G.L., Yokoyama, M.T., and Miller, E.R. (1990) Physiological relationships between microbiological status and dietary copper levels in the pig. *Journal of Animal Science* **68**: 1061-1071.

Siggers, R.H. Marshall, J.K., Shirkey, T.W., Drew, M.D., Laarveld, B. and Van Kessel, A.G. (2003) Cloning of porcine proglucagon and effect of commensal bacteria on relative expression in intestine of gnotobiotic pigs *Proceedings of the 9ᵗʰ International Symposium on the Digestive Physiology of Pigs.* **2**: 13-15.

Sharma, R., and Scumacher, U. (1995) Morphometric analysis of intestinal mucins under different dietary conditions and gut flora in rats. *Digestive Disease Science* **40**: 2532-2539.

Spurlock, M.E. (1997) Regulation of metabolism and growth during immune challenge: an overview of cytokine function. *Journal of Animal Science* **75**: 1773-1783.

Swords,W.E., Wu, C.C., Champlin, F.R., and Buddington, R.K. (1993) Postnatal changes in selected bacterial groups of the pig colonic microflora. *Biology of Neonates* **63**: 191-200.

Wostmann, B.S. (1996) *Germfree and gnotobiotic animal models: background and applications.* pp. 1-60. CRC Press, Boca Raton, FL.

Yokota, H., and Coates, M.E. (1982) The uptake of nutrients from the small intestine of gnotobiotic and conventional chicks. *British Journal of Nutrition* **47**: 349-356.

Regulation of gut function and immunity

Denise Kelly
Rowett Research Institute, Greenburn Road, Bucksburn, Aberdeen AB21 9SB, UK

Introduction

European-wide directives are now in place restricting the non-clinical use of production enhancers, chemotherapeutics and heavy metals in animal production. These legislative events have had a major impact on animal production within Europe and the UK, rendering current production systems inappropriate. Similarly in the US, the FDA are now actively promoting alternatives to feed-grade antibiotics. Hence, the animal industry worldwide is now faced with new and demanding challenges. From a practical standpoint, changes in weaning strategies, dietary regimes and rearing environments can be implemented in an attempt to accommodate the withdrawal of antibiotics. However, to address the wider issues of animal welfare, food safety, nutrient and mineral capture, in the context of both economic and environmental sustainability, animal production, once an applied science, needs to move to a more fundamental level.

Bacterial colonisation and immunity and disease resistance

Bacterial colonisation of gut surfaces

Adherence of bacteria to the intestinal mucosa remains a subject of great interest, primarily because the successful colonisation of micro-niches within the gut has been largely attributed to the ability to adhere and because attachment is recognised as an important initial event in the pathogenesis of bacterial infections. The mechanisms involved in bacterial attachment have been difficult to define primarily because the interaction involves a number of complex mechanisms including bacterial motility, chemotactic attraction and both specific and non-specific attachment to the mucus gel and epithelial surface.

61

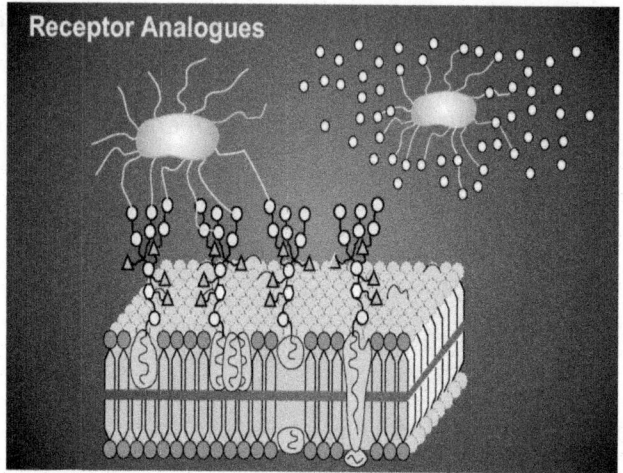

Figure 1.
Receptor
analogues and
competitive
exclusion effects
on gut bacteria.

Specific adhesion mechanisms can be advantageous to the host and bacterium. To the host, these mechanisms offer the advantage of promoting colonisation with commensal organisms that prevent the attachment of pathogenic micro-organisms. To the bacterium, adhesion offers the advantage of a firm attachment to tissue surfaces that can withstand the cleansing action of mucus flow, ciliary movement and peristalsis. Perhaps the greatest advantage, adhesion mechanisms allow the bacterium to attach to target tissues. Selective adhesion depends primarily upon the union of bacterial surface structures with complementary host structures called receptors. The adhesion of a particular species may vary considerably depending on host species, physiology, phenotype and tissue. It also appears that in virtually every system, bacteria employ more than one mechanism of binding.

Molecules involved in adhesion of bacteria to target cells

Lipotechoic acids, lipopolysaccharides (a family of toxic glycolipids present in the outer membrane of Gram negative bacteria), fimbrial adhesions and outer membrane proteins are all involved in gut wall interactions. Most of the adhesins reported thus far are proteins and fall in the category of lectins as defined by the capacity to bind specific sugar residues. Fimbrial adhesins are proteinaceous appendages of varying lengths and diameters, which protrude from the bacterial surface. The fimbriae are usually arranged around the bacterial cell wall, with 100's of fimbriae per bacterium. It is important to stress that bacterial adhesins are not always assembled into polymeric rods. For example, many adhesins cannot be visualised by standard electron microscopy (EM) and are thus considered to be non-fimbrial adhesins. The architecture of non-pilus adhesins is not well known but most are presumably linked to the cell surface as monomers or simple oligomers. In common the recognition of fimbrial and non-fimbrial adhesins is extremely fine-tuned allowing selective interactions with the host.

Type 1 and K88 fimbrial adhesions

Most Gram-negative bacteria possess fimbriae including *Escherichia coli*, Salmonella, Klebsiella, and Pseudomonas. Of the Gram positives Lactobacillus, Corynebacteria and Actinomyces have been shown to have filamentous appendages. *E. coli* is probably the most extensively studied group. This organism like many others has been found to express several different types of fimbriae, all with different adhesive properties. Type 1 fimbriae are found on the majority of *E. coli* strains. Enterotoxigenic strains of *E. coli* express other fimbrial types including K88, K99 and 987P or F6 Type 1 fimbriae, the subunits are tightly packed giving a rigid structure of approximately 7nm in diameter and approximately 2μm long. K88 fimbriae belong to another group and are thinner and flexible structures with a poorly defined diameter.

Chemically, fimbriae are protein polymers composed of identical subunits, with 1000 subunits per fimbriae. The molecular mass ranges between 15-30Kda. The subunits are held in stable thread-like structures via hydrophobic and electrostatic interactions. Fimbriae are tipped or interspersed with adhesive proteins. Classification of fimbriae was originally based on fimbrial diameter and the ability of different monosaccharides to inhibit red blood cell haemagglutination. However, stemming from fimbrial binding studies and inhibition experiments relevant receptor structures have been suggested for some adhesins.

Fimbriae are now classified according to their carbohydrate specificity. The specificity of a microbial fimbriae or lectin is defined in terms of the monosaccharide or oligosaccharide that most effectively inhibits the lectin induced agglutination or binding. Out of 100 microbial strains in which agglutinins have been found, more than 90% are bacteria with a pathogenic potential for higher organisms. Among bacterial species, the most thoroughly investigated group are the genus *E. coli* from which a wide variety of agglutinins have been isolated and identified e.g. K88 , K99, 987P, F41 these show diversity of carbohydrate specificity. The range of oligosaccharide structures which delineate specific receptor sites does not appear to be restrictive and indeed, available evidence suggests that colonisation may be optimised within animal species or even individuals of particular developmental status as determined by the availability of suitably defined receptor structures. For example, Type 1 fimbriae, which are the rigid structures, are often classified as to their whether haemagglutination can be inhibited by mannose, in which case they are designated as mannose sensitive. Those strains that are not inhibited by mannose are referred to as mannose resistant.

K99 *E. coli*, which cause diarrhoea in neonatal but not adult pigs, express fimbrial adhesins which bind N-glycoylneuraminyl-lactosyl-ceramide which is a sialylated ganglioside. This structure is present in abundance in newborn animals and rapidly declines in adults and may explain the susceptibility to infection.

Equally, K88 infection correlates with the expression of galactosylated structures although the precise receptor specificity is unknown. There is now evidence to suggest that the susceptibility to these pathogens could be due to the developmental window during which time the receptor is expressed. The range of specificities is confined to a limited number of structures, this is in part due to the fact that investigators have limited themselves to readily available oligosaccharide probes for inhibition experiments. Thus it should be expected that microbial lectins currently classified as specific for a certain structure may turn out to have significantly different specificities.

Figure 2.
K99 and rotavirus interactions with gut wall in young pigs.

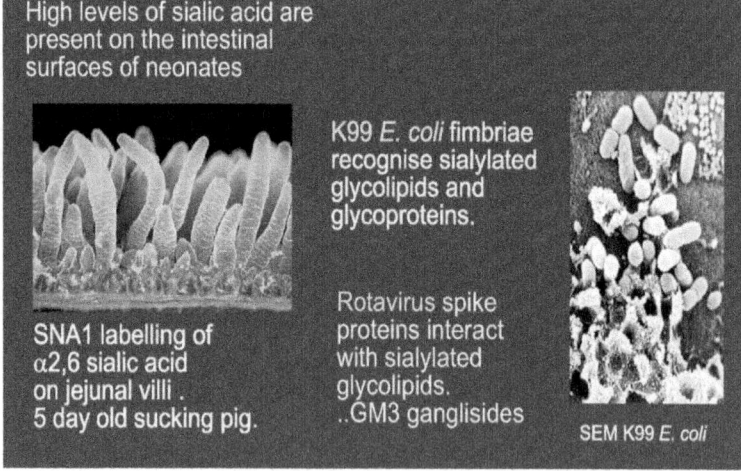

High levels of sialic acid are present on the intestinal surfaces of neonates

SNA1 labelling of α2,6 sialic acid on jejunal villi .
5 day old sucking pig.

K99 *E. coli* fimbriae recognise sialylated glycolipids and glycoproteins.

Rotavirus spike proteins interact with sialylated glycolipids.
..GM3 ganglisides

SEM K99 *E. coli*

Glycobiology and enteric infections

The molecules to which fimbriae bind are glycoconjugates. The surfaces of all cells are decorated with a complex array of sugar chains associated with glycoproteins and glycolipids, which extend from the surface of the epithelium and have been liken to mini bottle brushes. The structural diversity of oligosaccharides found on glycoproteins and glycolipids is theoretically enormous. Monosaccharides can be combined with each other in a variety of ways that differ not only in sequence and chain length but also in anomery (αß), position links and branching points. Hence, glycoconjugates exhibit considerable diversity in oligosaccharide sequences. Additionally, the oligosaccharides are not distributed uniformly among species, tissues and cells, hence the preferences of pathogens for specific host tissues.

The process, which adds oligosaccharides is referred to as glycosylation and is an important post-translational modification of structural and secretory glycoproteins.

Oligosaccharide structures are built up in a stepwise fashion during cellular differentiation; defined oligosaccharides are transferred one by one to developing oligosaccharide chains by a multienzyme glycosyltransferase system located in the membrane of the Golgi apparatus. Most glycoproteins carry oligosaccharide side chains N-glycosidically linked to amide nitrogen of asparagine and /or O-glycosidically linked to the hydroxl group of the amino acids serine and threonine. A diverse group of oligosaccharides are linked to lipids. In vertebrates most of these are glycosphingolipids, having hydrophilic oligosaccharide chain bound to a hydrophobic ceramide, which anchors the glycoconjugate to the membrane.

SNA recognises membrane sialylation i.e. α 2,6 sialylation. SNA binding decreases from newborn through to the weaned animal whereas ECA which recognises Gal-NacGlc increases, UEA fucosylated structures not present in the newborn intestine but increases in the suckled and weaned intestine and finally Maakia which recognises α 2,3 sialylation again increases dramatically in the suckling and weaning periods.

It is noteworthy that periods of microbial imbalance in neonates are associated with changes in epithelial glycosylation. This raises the question as to whether epithelial glycosylation can be used to predict disease susceptibility and identify periods of disease susceptibility?

K88 *E. coli* receptors

Galactose is a common constituent of O-linked glycans. Enterotoxigenic *E. coli* (ETEC) bearing K88 are frequently associated with out-breaks of diarrhoea in young pigs and are thought to recognise galactosyl residues although the precise specificity of this bacterium is unknown.

We, and others, have described a high molecular weight receptor complex in the intestines of weaned pigs. The receptor is expressed in the duodenum, jejunum and ileum. In K88 susceptible pigs, which developed the diarrhoea expression of a high molecular weight receptor complex was observed. K88 resistant pigs did not express this receptor. This result suggests that genetic differences in glycosyl moieties of the receptor complex provide the basis for disease susceptibility to K88ac ETEC. Recent investigations by Grange *et al.* (2002) show that the minimal carbohydrate structure needed for recognition by K88 adhesin variants contains HexNAc (GalNac or GlcNac) b-linked to a Gal residue. Significantly, Grange *et al.* (2002) also showed that modification of the HexNAc with fucose destroys adhesin-binding ability. Hence, the post-natal expression of fucosylated intestinal AO histo-blood antigens (King 1995, 2001) is therefore clearly implicated in the diminished susceptibility of older pigs to K88 ETEC infection. Similarly, the presence of a highly sialylated intestinal epithelial surface strongly influences the establishment of the enteric flora in young pigs. Many bacterial and viral pathogens have evolved adhesins that specifically bind to sialyl moieties and so facilitate enteric colonization. The sialic acids comprise a group of more than 40 acidic sugars. N-glycolylneuraminic acid (Neu5Gc) is one of the most common sialic acid types in the neonatal pig intestine (Malykh *et al.*, 2002). Neu5Gc-containing glycoconjugates play a crucial role in mediating infections by pathogens including K99 ETEC (Kyogoshima *et al.*, 1989; Teneberg *et al.*, 1990; Seignole *et al.*, 1991; Yuyama *et al.*, 1993), porcine rotavirus, (Rolsma *et al.*, 1998) and porcine transmissible gastroenteritis coronavirus (Schultze *et al.*, 1996). The biosynthesis and expression of Neu5Gc in the pig intestine declines markedly 2 weeks after birth (Malykh, 2002); again showing the strong link between mucosal glycosylation and the disease susceptibility of young pigs. These glycosylation events although partly pre-programmed are also sensitive to changes in dietary regime and the presence of selected commensal bacteria (Kelly and King, 1991; Kelly *et al.*, 1993; Bry *et al.*, 1996).

Oligosaccharides as receptor analogues

The host-microbe interface is currently in focus because of attempts to develop infection therapy based on natural receptor analogues. It is clearly recognised that a pre-requisite for the establishment of many enterobacterial infections including those caused by *E. coli* is the need for the pathogen to associate closely with host tissues. Intervention at this stage in the disease process is usually sufficient to suppress the development of clinical symptoms. This basic tenet has lead to the development of infection therapy based on natural receptor analogues or oligosaccharides. Multivalent ligands are more effective than free saccharides. This is particularly important for bacterial strains with multiple specificities were multivalent ligands may agglutinate the bacterial cell. For example, α Mannosyl glycoclusters have been shown to facilitate the development of high affinity inhibitors of the fimbrial lectin type 1.

Many potential natural sources of competing glycans exist. We have identified several competing receptor analogues from bovine milk that are capable of completly blocking the attachment of K88 *E. coli* to the intestine of susceptible pigs.

Bacterial attachment/crosstalk and innate immunity

Very little information exists describing the development, function and activation of cells of the innate immune system. These cells, which function independent of prior exposure to bacterial antigens, provide first line defense and are extremely important in early life when the adaptive immune system is functionally immature. Epithelial cells are now recognised to play a major role in innate immunity, forming a highly specialised physical and functional barrier to dietary and microbial antigens. By virtue of tight junctions, epithelial cells provide a physical barrier to lumenal antigen; they also actively secrete mucin and anti-microbial peptides that limit bacterial attachment and invasion of the epithelium but, also secrete bi-directionally, cytokines and chemokines that alter both epithelial and lymphoid cell function. Each of these characteristics are crucial for host defence but their development in pig gut epithelial cells and importantly, the influence of microbial colonisation, environment, weaning age and diet are currently undefined.

Epithelial cells also respond directly to colonising bacteria. They utilise specific cell-surface pattern recognition receptors to detect and respond to the presence of bacteria and specific bacterial moeities. A number of diverse receptor systems are expressed on epithelial cell surfaces that recognise bacteria and communicate signals to underlying lymphoid cell populations.

Toll-like receptors–bacterial detectors

Toll-like receptors (TLRs) are emerging as a functionally important class of membrane receptors that also play a key role in bacterial recognition. TLRs recognise conserved molecular patterns (pathogen-associated molecular patterns, PAMPs) and (commensal-associated molecular patterns, CAMPs) shared by large groups of bacteria and other gut micro-organisms. TLR expression has not to date been investigated in the pig but specific gene sequences have been identified (Kelly, unpublished). TLRs are expressed on both

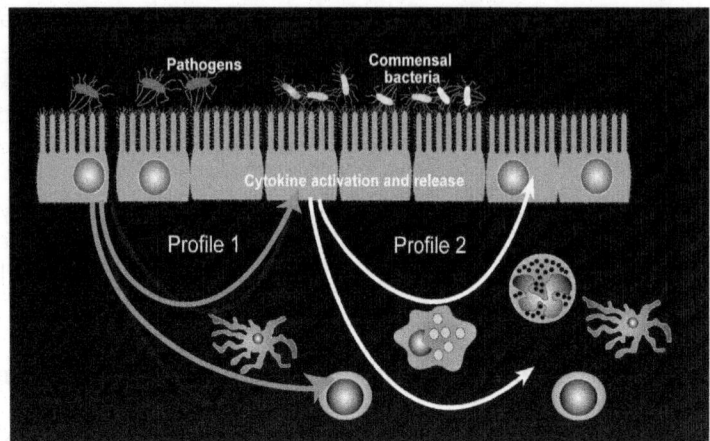

Figure 3. Cellular mechanisms of bacterial/ mucosal crosstalk.

epithelial and lymphoid cells and, in addition to their important function in bacterial ligand recognition, they also activate signal transduction pathways (e.g. Nuclear factor kappa B [NFκB] and mitogen activated protein kinases [MAPkinases]) that trigger gene expression, that via both autocrine and paracrine mechanisms alter epithelial and lymphoid cell function. Currently, in humans there are eleven known TLRs; of these, the ligands for TLR 2, 3 , 4, 5 and 9 have been identified. Some TLRs appear to respond to only one PAMP, such as TLR5, which is activated by the bacterial protein flagellin (Hayashi *et al.*, 2001) and TLR9 that is activated by CpG bacterial DNA (Bauer *et al.*, 2001). Other TLRs however, appear to be more promiscuous with several PAMPs having been reported to produce pro-inflammatory responses *via* activation of either TLR2 or TLR4 (reviewed in Akira *et al.*, 2001). TLR development and regulation in response to bacterial colonisation has not yet been addressed in the pig intestine and only to a very limited extent in rodents. Furthermore, TLRs are transducing receptors and hence the autocrine and paracrine impact of TLR ligation and gene expression, on the function of epithelial and underlying lymhoid cells is also poorly defined.

The importance of TLRs in pathogen clearance and resolution of disease

A number of bacterial pathogens that infect intestinal tissues have been shown to induce strong Th1 responses in humans and in mice. Recent data from several sources have shown that both interleukin 12 (IL12) and gamma interferon (IFNγ), which favour the differentiation of Th1 cells, are important cytokines in limiting intracellular bacterial infections (Simmons *et al.*, 2002). It is also recognised, that whilst T cells are vital in bacterial clearance they also mediate much of the tissue pathology associated with infection thereby implicating the host immune response as a major cause of tissue pathology (Vallance *et al.*, 2002). However, many of the pathogens commonly encountered in human and animal infections induce self-limiting diseases suggesting that bacterial/host mechanisms have evolved that minimise disease severity, tissue pathology, morbidity and host mortality. Recent data from our laboratory, and others, supports the hypothesis that TLRs that recognise molecular structures shared among bacterial pathogens may, in addition to contributing to pathogen clearance *via* innate and adaptive immunity, also facilitate the resolution of immune responses thereby preventing or reducing the likelihood of chronic or lethal infection.

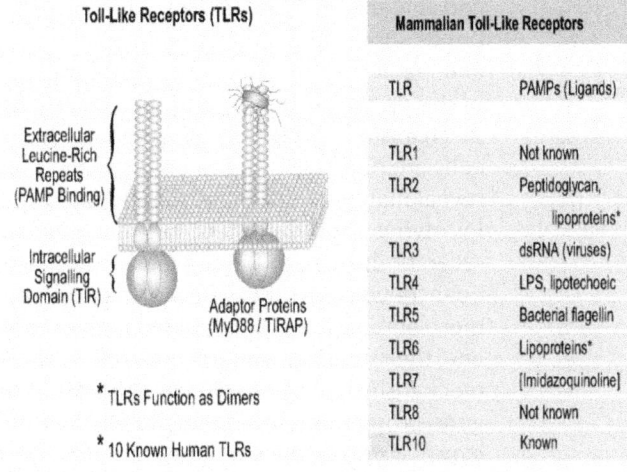

Figure 4.
Toll-like receptors
in mammals.

TLR	PAMPs (Ligands)
TLR1	Not known
TLR2	Peptidoglycan,
	lipoproteins*
TLR3	dsRNA (viruses)
TLR4	LPS, lipotechoeic
TLR5	Bacterial flagellin
TLR6	Lipoproteins*
TLR7	[Imidazoquinoline]
TLR8	Not known
TLR10	Known

Consistent with the above hypothesis that germ-line TLR receptors, in addition to triggering innate and adaptive immunity, are critical to the resolution of immune responses, TLRs have been shown to induce both pro-inflammatory and anti-inflammatory gene expression (Ronni *et al.*, 2003). Furthermore, defects in TLRs have been documented to increase the susceptibility to pathogens and sepsis syndrome (Lorenz *et al.*, 2002; Hawn *et al.*, 2003) and also have been linked to chronic inflammatory diseases (Zuany-Amorim *et al.*, 2002).

It is our hypothesis that effective host immunity to gut pathogens is critically-dependent upon appropriate TLR activation and signalling and, that resolution of the host response is an inherent (self) feature of these receptors, achieved in part, by divergence in downstream gene expression. We propose that TLRs display dual functionality and that this biological property accounts for both their pro-inflammatory (bacterial killing) and protective functions (resolution of the host immune response and maintenance of tissue integrity). Finally, we propose that divergent signalling and gene expression downstream of TLR receptor results in factors that influence epithelial function and integrity and can promote the expression of distinct protective T cell subsets.

Adaptive immunity and tolerance

Intestinal cells and M cells

Intestinal epithelial cells and M cells provide the first point of contact with intestinal bacteria. The interactions between bacteria, M cells and epithelial cells are now of major interest as the weight of evidence builds supporting a dynamic interaction which, through autocrine and paracrine mechanisms, profoundly influences the function of the epithelial barrier and the underlying lymphoid tissues. The mechanism by which bacteria modulate gene expression in epithelial cells are just beginning to be unravelled, but already many studies reveal highly evolved and sophisticated systems of communication involving modulation of cellular events from the level of the receptor through to the nucleus. Previously, much of this work has been devoted to the study of pathogens, however, increasingly more emphasis is now directed to the study of commensal bacteria and their mechanisms of interaction. Irrespective of the precise mechansims, it is now clear that bacteria can upregulate a complex gene programme in epithelial cells and by doing so influence the expression of a diverse array of epithelial products drammatically altering the biochemistry, physiology and function of the intestinal barrier. As our understanding of the mechanisms of interaction between commensal bacteria and gut cells increases concomitantly, the potential for beneficial manipulation and modulation of the gut response increases.

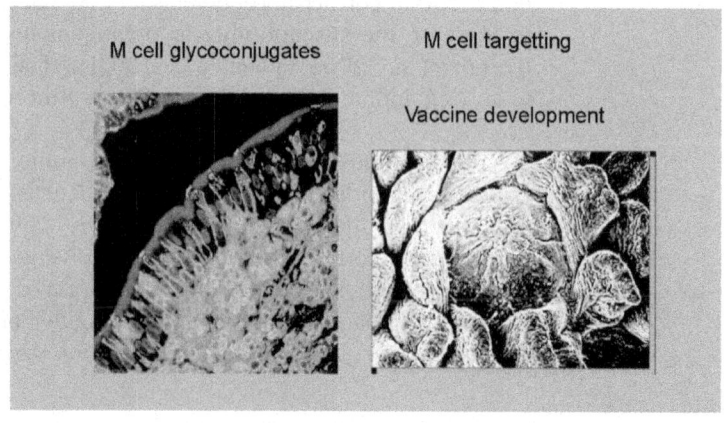

Figure 5.
M cells - immune defence mechanisms.

Dendritic cells and bacterial antigens

Activation of adaptive immune responses begins with processing and presentation of antigen by professional antigen presenting cells (APCs). Dendritic cells (DCs) represent a key antigen-presenting cell and are important for development of innate and adaptive immunity. In the pig virtually nothing is known about the development, differentiation, function, activation and recruitment of DCs and how these individual processes are influenced by nutrition and mucosal colonisation.

Similarly, phenotypic studies strongly suggest that the mucosal immune system remains relatively immature throughout the "normal commercial weaning" period. Taken together with the well-recognised decline in passively transferred maternal antibody at this time, this data highlights the vulnerability of the early-weaned piglet (Bailey and Stokes, 2003). The factors involved in promoting APC and T cell function and the development of specific T cell subsets (e.g. regulatory T cells) are poorly defined.

Novel approaches to gut health

Microbial diversity and development of immunity

Colonisation of the intestine with microflora is essential for the normal development of humoral and cellular responses (Hooper and Gordon, 2001). Studies in germ-free piglets have highlighted the importance of an intestinal microflora on the phased development of the mucosal immune system (Rothkotter et al., 1991; Pabst et al., 1988: Barman et al., 1997). The gut is sterile at birth and is then colonised by microbes from the mother and environment. Gut microflora participates in health maintenance by forming a barrier preventing gut invasion by pathogenic bacteria, a phenomenon known as colonisation resistance (Rolfe, 1997). Although much emphasis has been placed on the role of bifidobacteria and lactobacilli (less than 1% of the normal colonic flora) in maintaining gut health and barrier function and for stimulating a healthy immune function, other prevalent bacterial species are emerging as potentially important candidates (e.g. Gram-negative Cytophaga-Flavobacteria-Bacteroides cluster and Gram-positive Clostridial clusters XIVa and IV). By combining microbial profiling (microarray based 16S ribotyping) with functional studies defining the responses of specific gut cell populations (epithelial and lymphoid) to colonising bacteria it may be possible to identify important microbial species with immune-potentiating/modulating properties. Colonisation by a single bacterial species has already been illustrated to trigger significant phenotypic and functional maturation in specific lymphoid cell populations. Knowledge of the microbes and microbial antigens that specifically potentiate both the development of the epithelial barrier and the function of innate/adaptive arms (DCs and T cells) of the immune sytem is not currently available.

Novel molecular techniques provide a unique opportunity for investigating bacterial diversity along the gut (Flint *et al.*, 1999; Mackie *et al.*, 1998, Simpson *et al.*, 1999). Based on 16S rDNA sequences, research at the Rowett (Pryde *et al.*, 1999) has shown that the majority of bacteria closely associated with the gut wall are unrelated to known organisms. Valuable information on immune development can therfore be derived from molecular profiling studies which factor in important environmental (microbial) and dietary variables.

Impact of microbial colonisation on adaptive immune responses

Currently, our understanding of the mechanisms by which microbial colonisation potentiates immune development and modulates the adaptive immune response is poor. Unravelling the responses generated towards bacterial antigens against a complex background of colonising flora which actively modulate the host response represents a significant challenge. It is likely that even within the complex ecosystem of the gut, dominant bacterial antigens direct and determine the immune response. Certain bacterial components such as flagellin are recognised to be highly immunogenic but are also potent immune-modulators. The combined effect of these molecules must profoundly influence immune outcome.

TLRs and modulation of innate/adaptive immunity

Studies undertaken at the Rowett investigating the signalling pathways induced in epithelial cells following exposure to commensal and pathogenic bacteria, have shown that both bacterial groups can induce TLR-mediated ativation of NF-κB and MAPkinase signalling pathways. It can therefore be concluded that both commensal and pathogenic bacteria appear to possess molecular patterns that recognise and activate TLR receptors expressed on epithelial cells. Importantly, we have found that certain strains of bacteria can regulate the host cellular responses, by differential modulation of host cell signal transduction pathways and by influencing nuclear transcription events (Kelly *et al.*, 2004). This modulation can be induced with bacterially-derived products generated by live bacteria following contact with epithelial cells. That such bacterial-derived products get beyond the epithelium to regulate cells of the adaptive immune system is also a strong possibility and hence their direct impact on adaptive immunity is also important. Finally, the existence of potent immuno-modulators and immuno-stimulants, either secreted or surface-bound, on colonising bacteria is certain; identifying such components and defining their mode of action would provide novel targets and strategies for promoting natural immune defence mechanisms during postnatal development.

Genomic analysis of the gut immune system

Much of the mechanistic studies on immune development and modulation have utilised mice. Few mechanistic studies on immune function have been undertaken in pigs or indeed other domestic species, and as a consequence much of the sequence information describing important immunological proteins is not currently available (e.g. pig sequences for TLRs). The application of genomic strategies provides an unparalleled opportunity to unveil important biological effects triggered by gut microbes on the early development of the innate and adaptive immune systems. Such genomic approaches will be screened for differentially-regulated genes by quantitative expression analyses of tissues and cells derived from conventional-reared animals under defined conditions.

References

Akira, S., Takeda, K. and Kaisho, T. (2001) Toll-like receptors: critical proteins linking innate and acquired immunity. *Nature Immunology* **2**: 675-680.

Barman, N.N., Bianchi, A.T., Zwart, R.J., Pabst, R. and Rothkotter, H.J. (1997) Jejunal and ileal Peyer's patches in pigs differ in their postnatal development. *Anatomy and Embryology (Berlin).* **195(1)**: 41-50.

Bry, L., Falk, P.G., Midtvedt, T. and Gordon, J.I. (1996) A model of host-microbial interactions in an open mammalian ecosystem. *Science.* **273(5280)**: 1380-1383.

Grange, P.A., Mouricout M.A., Levery S.B., Francis D.H., and Erickson A.K. (2002) Evaluation of receptor binding specificity of *Escherichia coli* K88 (F4) fimbrial adhesin variants using porcine serum transferrin and glycosphingolipids as model receptors. *Infection and Immunity* **70(5)**: 2336-2343.

Hawn,T.R., Verbon, A., Lettinga, K.D., Zhao, L.P., Li, S.S., Laws, R.J., Skerrett, S.J., Beutler, B., Schroeder, L., Nachman, A., Ozinsky, A., Smith, K.D. and Aderem, A. (2003) A common dominant TLR5 stop codon polymorphism abolishes flagellin signaling and i s associated with susceptibility to legionnaires' disease. *Journal of Experimental Medicine* **198**: 1563-1572.

Hayashi, F., Smith, K.D., Ozinsky, A., Hawn, T.R., Yi, E.C., Goodlett, D.R., Eng, J.K., Akira, S., Underhill, D.M., and Aderem, A. (2001) The innate immune response to bacterial flagellin is mediated by Toll-like receptor 5. *Nature* **410**: 1099-1103.

Hooper, L.V., and Gordon, J.I. (2001) Glycans as legislators of host-microbial interactions: spanning the spectrum from symbiosis to pathogenicity. *Glycobiology* **11(2)**: 1R-10R.

Kelly, D., and King, T.P. (2001) A review – luminal bacteria and regulation of gut function and immunity. In: *Manipulating Pig Production VIII*. Edited by Cranwell, P.D. pp. 263-276. Australasian Pig Science Association, Australia .

Kelly, D., Begbie, R., and King, T.P. (1994) Nutritional influences on interactions between bacteria and the small intestinal mucosa. *Nutrition Research Reviews* **7**: 233-257.

Kelly, D., Campbell, J.I., King, T.P., Grant, G., Jansson, E.A., Coutts, A.G.P., Pettersson, S., and Conway, S. (2004) Commensal anaerobic gut bacteria attenuate inflammation by regulating nuclear-cytoplasmic shuttling of PPAR and RelA. *Nature Immunology* In press.

King, T.P., Begbie, R., Slater, D., McFadyen, M., Thom, A., and Kelly, D. (1995) Sialylation of intestinal microvillar membranes of newborn, sucking and weaned pigs. *Glycobiology* **5**: 525-534.

Kyogashima, M., Ginsburg, V., and Krivan, H.C. (1989) Escherichia coli K99 binds to N-glycolylsialoparagloboside and N-glycolyl-GM3 found in piglet small intestine. *Archives of Biochemistry and Biophysics* **270(1)**: 391-397.

Jeyasingham, M.D., Butty, P., King, T.P., Begbie, R., a nd Kelly, D. (1999) *Escherichia coli* K88 receptor expression in intestine of disease-susceptible weaned pigs. *Veterinary Microbiology* **68:** 219-234.

Lorenz, E., Mira, J.P., Frees, K.L., and Schwartz, D.A. (2002) Relevance of mutations in the TLR4 receptor in patients with Gram-negative septic shock. *Archives of Internal Medicine.* **162:** 1028-1032.

Malykh, Y.N., King, T.P., Logan, E., Kelly, D., Schauer, R., and Shaw, L. (2003) Regulation of N-glycolylneuraminic acid biosynthesis in developing pig small intestine. *Biochemical Journal* **370(Pt 2)**: 601-607.

Pabst, R., Geist, M., Rothkötter, H.J., and Fritz, F.J. (1988) Postnatal development and lymphocyte production of jejunal and ileal Peyer's patches in normal and gnotobiotic pigs. *Immunology* **64**: 539-544.

Pryde, S.E., Richardson, A.J., Stewart, C.S., and Flint, H.J. (1999) Molecular analysis of the microbial diversity present in the colonic wall, colonic lumen, and cecal lumen of a pig. *Applied and Environmental Microbiology* **65(12)**: 5372-5377.

Rolsma, M.D., Kuhlenschmidt, T.B., Gelberg, H.B., and Kuhlenschmidt, M.S. (1998) Structure and function of a ganglioside receptor for porcine rotavirus. *Journal of Virology* **72(11)**: 9079-9091.

Ronni, T., Agarwal, V., Haykinson, M., Haberland, M.E., Cheng, G., and Smale, S.T. (2003) Common interaction surfaces of the toll-like receptor 4 cytoplasmic domain stimulate multiple nuclear targets. *Molecular and Cellular Biology* **23**: 2543-2555.

Rothkotter, H.J., Ulbrich, H., and Pabst, R. (1991) The postnatal development of gut lamina propria lymphocytes: number, proliferation, and T and B cell subsets in conventional and germ-free pigs. *Pediatric Research* **29**: 237-242.

Schultze, B., Krempl, C., Ballesteros, M.L., Shaw, L., Schauer, R., Enjuanes, L., and Herrler G. (1996) Transmissible gastroenteritis coronavirus, but not the related porcine respiratory coronavirus, has a sialic acid (N-glycolylneuraminic acid) binding activity. *Journal of Virology* . **70(8)**: 5634-7563.

Seignole, D., Mouricout, M., Duval-Iflah, Y., Quintard, B., and Julien, R. (1991) Adhesion of K99 fimbriated Escherichia coli to pig intestinal epithelium: correlation of adhesive and non-adhesive phenotypes with the sialoglycolipid content. *Journal of General Microbiology* **137** (7): 1591-1601.

Simmons, C.P., Goncalves, N.S., Ghaem-Maghami, M., Bajaj-Elliott, M., Clare, S., Neves, B., Frankel, G., Dougan, G., and MacDonald,T.T. (2002) Impaired resistance and enhanced pathology during infection with a noninvasive, attaching-effacing enteric bacterial pathogen, Citrobacter rodentium, in mice lacking IL-12 or IFN-gamma. *Journal of Immunology* **168**: 1804-1812 .

Simpson, J.M., McCracken, V.J., White, B.A., Gaskins, H.R., and Mackie, R.I. (1999) Application of denaturant gradient gel electrophoresis for the analysis of the porcine gastrointestinal microbiota. *Journal of Microbiological Methods* **36(3)**: 167-179.

Teneberg, S., Willemsen, P., de Graaf, F.K. and Karlsson, K.A. (1990) Receptor-active glycolipids of epithelial cells of the small intestine of young and adult pigs in relation to susceptibility to infection with Escherichia coli K99. *FEBS Letters* **263(1)**: 10-14.

Vallance, B.A., Deng, W., Knodler, L.A., and Finlay, B.B. (2002) Mice lacking T and B lymphocytes develop transient colitis and crypt hyperplasia yet suffer impaired bacterial clearance during Citrobacter rodentium infection. *Infection and Immunity* **70**: 2070-2081.

Yuyama, Y., Yoshimatsu, K., Ono, E., Saito, M., and Naiki, M. (1993) Postnatal change of pig intestinal ganglioside bound by Escherichia coli with K99 fimbriae. *Journal of Biochemistry (Tokyo)* **113(4)**: 488-492.

Zuany-Amorim, C., and Hastewell, J. (2002) Toll-like receptors as potential therapeutic targets for multiple diseases. *Nature Reviews Drug Discovery* **1**: 797-807.

Controlling gastrointestinal disease to improve absorptive membrane integrity and optimize digestion efficiency

Stephen R Collett
The University of Georgia, Athens, Georgia, USA

Introduction

Many broiler and turkey producers are withdrawing growth-promoting antibiotics in response to retailer and consumer demand. Antibiotics have been an integral part of poultry feed for the past 50 years (Rosen, 1995) and decades of research and field use have established their efficiency as growth promoters or more correctly, 'pronutrients' (Rosen, 1995; Rosen, 1996a).

In-feed antibiotics have been shown to enhance performance through subtly changing the composition of the normal flora (Rosen, 1995; Anderson *et al.*, 2000). Much of the defining research in this regard was completed prior to the mid 1980s (Anderson *et al.*, 2000). The complexities of the industry have changed considerably in the last 20 years and currently antibiotics are included in meat bird rations primarily to suppress specific pathogens associated with known diseases, such as *Clostridium perfringens*.

In contrast to the direct bacteriostatic or bacteriocidal activity of the gram-positive antibiotics, the alternatives thus far studied often have little if any direct effect on these gram-positive organisms. With the withdrawal of antibiotic growth promoters, clostridial infections with consequential losses from increased mortality and reduced feed conversion efficiency and quality have become a primary concern.

Clostridial enterotoxaemias

Stress that is induced by climatic or management factors leads to a disturbance in the composition of intestinal flora, resulting in selective growth and synthesis of toxins by various Clostridium spp. During the past five years enterotoxemia has resulted in the following conditions:

- Necrotic enteritis: characterized by mild to severe enteritis that occurs from 14 days through to flock depletion. Losses are attributed to acute mortality that may affect 37% of the flock, depressed growth rate and lowered feed conversion efficiency (Wages and Opengart, 2003b).

- Cholangiohepatitis: an emerging condition in broilers results from an ascending infection from the duodenum, affecting the major bile ducts and gall bladder. Affected flocks show degraded performance and a high proportion of livers is condemned at processing (Sasaki *et al.*, 2000).

- Gangrenous dermatitis occurs most frequently when vast numbers of *Clostridium perfringens* spores accumulate in the litter. Superficial dermal lacerations become infected and the ensuing gangrenous dermatitis rapidly develops into cellulitis and gangrenous myofascitis, resulting in acute death and increased condemnation (Wages and Opengart, 2003).

- Botulism is an emerging and often misdiagnosed condition in broilers, characterized by paresis and paralysis. The condition is frequently confused with lameness due to the skeletal abnormalities it causes. Losses of up to 10% have been recorded in flocks (Martinez and Wobester, 1999; Wobester, 1997).

Pathogenesis of clostridial enterotoxaemias

The development of clostridial infections and resulting enterotoxemia is primarily the result of toxin production (Barnes, 2003). These normally innocuous members of the gut flora become pathogenic in the presence of a range of intrinsic and extrinsic stressors, which enhance proliferation and toxin production. Abnormal proliferation of Clostridia in the intestinal tract occurs in birds that have a compromised immune response, or unstable gastrointestinal environment (Figure 1).

The most common precursors of infection include damage to the intestinal mucosa, change in dietary composition and inappropriate management of feeding, watering, heating, cooling and ventilation systems. It is however more likely a combination of factors that precipitate the disease (Kaldhusdal and Skjevre, 1996), as follows:

- Damage to the intestinal mucosa as a consequence of intestinal infections, with coccidiosis as the predominant initiator of necrotic enteritis. Low-grade *Eimeria acervulina* and *E. maxima* result in a transitory decrease in intestinal motility and altered passage time of digesta approximately 5 days after infection (Wages and Opengart, 2003). Concurrently there is leakage of protein from damaged enterocytes and a change in pH which favours multiplication of *Clostridium perfringens*.

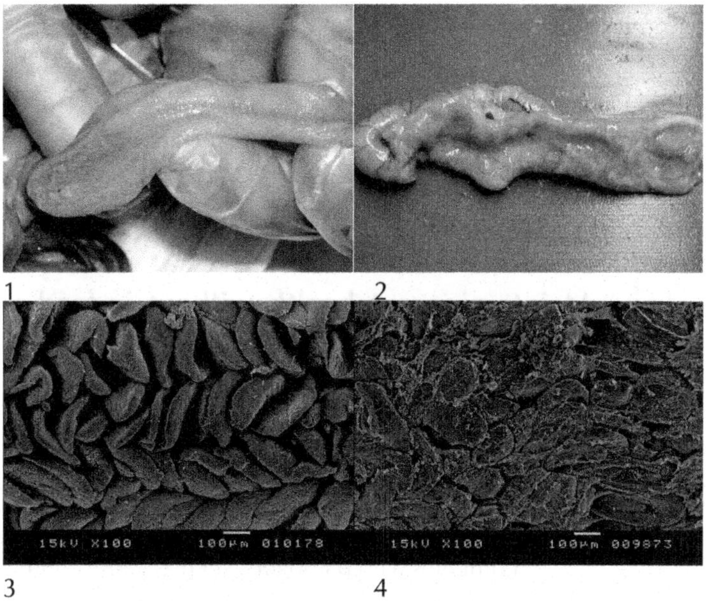

Figure 1. Gut showing damage to internal surface (2) and villi (4) versus normal health tissue (1 and 3).

- Change in feed composition including the introduction of animal by-products or substitution of wheat and barley for corn, resulting in an increase in the viscosity of digesta, delayed passage rate, and an alteration in the composition of intestinal flora (Branton *et al.*, 1987; Kaldusdal and Hofshagen, 1997; Johnson and Pinedo, 1971).

- Immuno-suppression caused by systemic infections including infectious bursal disease, Marek's disease and chick anemia are well-known disease entities that predispose flocks to clostridial infections (Lukert and Saif, 2003; Schat, 2003; Whitter and Schat, 1997). There are however several other causes of immune suppression including mycotoxin poisoning (Hoerr, 2003) and stress (Siegel, 1994) that pose significant risk in today's intensive production systems. Stress resulting from inappropriate management of the house environment is currently one of the most frequently encountered predispositions.

  - Overstocking, resulting in deterioration of litter quality and competition for access to feeders and drinkers.
  - Saturation of the litter due to malfunction or improper operation of ventilation systems.
  - Starvation associated with delays in feed delivery or breakdown of feeding systems, including transfer augers, chains and drive motors.

- Initiation of meal feeding programs for broilers and restricted feeding for replacement breeder pullets.
- Disturbance associated with manual vaccination, weighing or partial depletion ('thinning') of flocks.

Although growth-promoting antibiotics which suppress Clostridium spp compensate for deficiencies in management and control of disease, alternative preventive programs are required, to sustain organic production and for countries where the use of antibiotics is restricted or in disfavour.

Maintaining gut health without in-feed antibiotic growth promoters

To establish an effective gut health program without antibiotics it is important to consider all possible areas of intervention and the program focus should be to optimize gastrointestinal absorptive membrane development and integrity. The early establishment and maintenance of a beneficial intestinal flora is key since the gut flora competes with pathogens such as Clostridium spp. and a favourable flora also helps to stimulate early enterocyte development.

The basis of a gut health program is to protect flock health by establishing and maintaining a stable normal flora as soon after hatch as possible. This approach provides several options for intervention:

1. Seed the gut with a host-adapted favourable flora to accelerate the development of a climax flora.

2. Prepare a favourable gastrointestinal environment for

   a. the rapid establishment of a favourable and stable climax gut flora.
   b. rapid enterocyte development to accelerate maturation of gut, digestion efficiency and absorption capacity

3. Exclude pathogens to maintain the stability of the gut flora by

   a. gut flora management to enhance competitive exclusion
   b. pathogen blocking
   c. immune modulation
   d. preventing the negative impact of mycotoxins on the gut flora

4. Enhance resilience through immune modulation

5. Decrease passage of intact nutrients by improving digestion and absorption to prevent protein and energy through-flow to the

lower gastro-intestinal tract and avoid the negative impact that this has on the gut flora profile.

a. improving membrane integrity
b. improving nutrient availability

While the first step in such a gut health management program is to prevent unfavourable flora communities from colonizing the gut the extent of an appropriate intervention program is dependent on the degree of challenge.

Strategies to manage gut health

In response to the need for alternatives to in-feed antibiotics research and development effort has focused on the quest for effective replacements as indicated by the plethora of performance enhancers making an appearance on the world market. Although there is growing scientific support for many of these replacements (Rosen, 2003; Hooge, 2003a, 2003b) the claim of efficacy is in many cases inadequately substantiated (Rosen, 2003).

An effective product should have a significant and sustainable beneficial impact on animal production and health, be proven safe for both the animal and human population, be easy to apply and store and provide a substantial return on investment (Collett and Dawson, 2001). An average improvement of 2.26% in FCR and 1.41% in weight gain in 74% of the cases has been established as the standard by decades of antibiotic use and research (Rosen, 2003). This data and years of field use provide the potential user with a certain degree of confidence.

Perceived failure of antibiotic replacements to satisfy expectations for equivalence to antibiotics in the field has increased industry scepticism and reduced the credibility of research on these products. The search has been for a single intervention or product to replace antibiotics and this has slowed progress. It has become increasingly clear that a multi-factorial approach is needed. A number of options are available for enhancing the performance of poultry in the absence of specific in-feed antibiotics. To be successful an alternative strategy or program must yield comparable economic return and production efficiency must be sustainable.

Seeding the gut with favourable microflora

a. Parent flock microflora management

Since most normal eggs have a sterile surface prior to oviposition the point of lay is the first major opportunity for contamination. The level of contamination varies from $10^3 - 10^5$ cfu. per egg in clean conditions and $10^7 - 10^8$ cfu per egg under dirty conditions thus confirming that contamination is a function of the environment into which the egg is laid (Board and Fuller, 1994). These eggshell contaminants provide the first seed stock for chick and poult gut colonization at hatch. Positive manipulation of parent flock flora provides the first opportunity for offspring flora management. Bio-Mos used to positively alter the normal flora in parent flocks has been shown to significantly enhance chick resistance to pathogen colonization (Fernandez *et al.*, 2001) (Figure 2).

Figure 2. Effect of mannose and mannan-oligosaccharide on caecal colonisation of 1-10 d broilers challenged with hen caecal conents (Fernandez *et al.*, 2001).

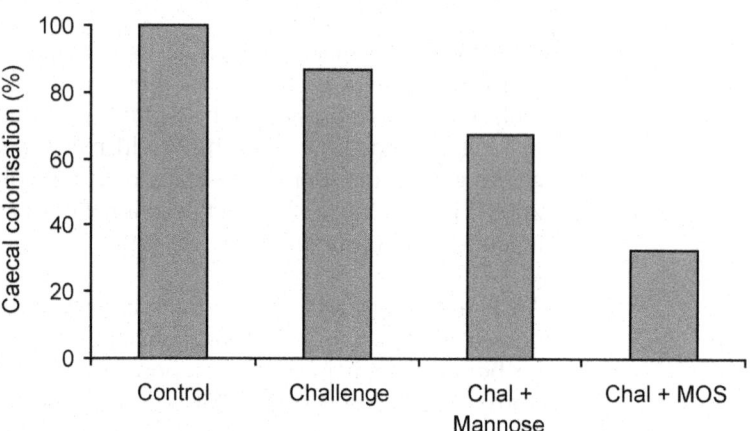

b.   **Direct fed microbial application**

Lactobacillus acidophilus and *Streptococcus faecium* have shown promise in reducing the impact of low-grade necrotic enteritis on performance when used as a direct-fed microbial. The only published report in which an alternative matches an antibiotic in protecting against necrotic enteritis induced mortality is that of Hofacre *et al.* (2003). In this study the combination of a direct-fed microbial (All-Lac XCL™) and mannoprotein (Bio-Mos™) were shown to be comparable to 50g per ton of Bacitracin-MD. This study also suggests that the degree of protection elicited by a direct fed microbial may be strain specific since, as with previous studies *Lactobacillus acidophilus* and *Streptococcus faecium* were the two primary organisms used.

c.   **House flora management**

While it is possible to change the composition of the *gut flora* reasonably quickly (within the first cycle) it takes several grow-out cycles to change the profile of the house flora. The house flora profile changes as a result of replacement and or displacement of the house flora with the gut flora. Since the gut flora of the birds raised during the previous 3-5 grow-out cycles determines the composition of the house flora at the next placement it is important to adopt a methodical, progressive and carefully designed program to successfully manage the composition of the house flora.

The logistics and cost of long-term experimentation has forced researchers to neglect testing the long-term effects of pronutrient programs. Although there are literally thousands of pronutrient trials demonstrating their efficacy or lack thereof, the literature is devoid of data showing the long-term effect of such programs. Single point evaluation gives no indication of the influence that an intervention has in a continuous production system.

Gut flora determines the composition of the litter/house flora (Lilijebjelke *et al.*, 2003) that in turn acts as the seed stock for the gut flora of the next placement. While the use of a pronutrient can alter the gut flora within a couple of weeks it takes several grow-out cycles to change the house flora (Avellaneda *et al.*, 2003; Idris *et al.*, 2003; Lilijebjelke *et al.*,2003; Schildknecht, *et al.*, 2003a; 2003b) Although recently reported this is by no means a new concept. Both rotation and shuttle programs have been used for decades.

Preparing the gastrointestinal environmental

Meta analysis (Partanen and Mroz, 1999) and literature review (Partanen, 2001) indicate that water and feed acidification have an important role to play in gut flora management. While these reviews indicate that organic acids and their salts have potential as alternatives to antibiotics in pig nutrition the case for acidification of poultry feed and water is less convincing (Rosen, 2003; Collett and Dawson, 2001). The pronutrient potential of commercial acid preparations is thought to arise from the antibacterial effects of their ionization properties. Acid ionization varies considerably according to type, concentration and mix of acids used and is further modified by the pH, buffering capacity and water activity of the feed, water and gut content (Chung and Goeffert, 1970). Since their activity in the gastrointestinal tract is so variable, systematic studies of the effects of a variety of acidifiers are not available. It is not possible to determine the overall responses to complex acidification strategies or to compare these with antibiotic supplementation strategies using objective analytical process (Rosen, 2003).

Organic acids, which include fatty acids, volatile fatty acids (VFA) lipophylic acids or carboxylic acids are designated as organic because of the presence of a carboxyl group (-COOH). Early research on the antibacterial activity of organic acids has focused on the short chain monocarboxcylic acids but derivatives of this group are equally important. The more important derivatives include the unsaturated (sorbic), hydroxylic (citric, lactic) phenolic (salacylic) and multicarboxylic (citric) acids.

The low molecular-weight acids are liquid at room temperature and while the short chain acids (C_{1-6}) are miscible with water the medium chain acids (C_{7-10}) readily form salts that are soluble in water. As chain length increases so to does the volatility but when considering feed addition this becomes an important consideration. Preconditioning and pelleting temperatures are in the region of 82-85°C, which is in excess of the boiling point of even the less volatile salts of these organic acids.

The dissociation of an organic acid in solution is predictable and in accordance with the Henderson-Hassebach equation. The extent to which the acid dissociates is dependant on the affinity of the carboxyl group for its proton (H^+) and is expressed as its dissociation constant (K_a or $pK_a = -logK_a$). The higher the pK_a value the stronger the molecules affinity for protons. Organic acids have a relatively high dissociation constant and are thus relatively reluctant proton donors in aqueous solution and thus weak acids. Dissociation of a weak acid is pH dependent. This is in contrast to strong inorganic acids, which have very low pK_a values and consequently very readily donate protons (H^+) even at low pH.

Comparative evaluation of the antibacterial activity of different organic acids is notoriously difficult. There are no standardized testing procedures and since the degree of dissociation is dependent on the pK_a value it is only possible to compare acids that have the same pK_a values. In addition to pH, the buffering capacity of the medium, acid concentration and structure and the presence of the acid salt or other organic acids will all affect the antibacterial activity.

Excluding pathogens

In order for most bacteria to colonize the gastrointestinal tract they first need to attach to the epithelial surface. They do this via carbohydrate projections such as lectins that recognize certain epithelial surface sugars. Many enteric pathogens attach to these sugars via Type 1 fimbriae, which recognize mannose. Bio-Mos blocks pathogen attachment and hence colonization by occupying the lectin attachment site on type 1 fimbriae.

The term 'competitive exclusion' is used to describe the inability of one population of micro-organisms to colonise the gut because of the presence of another population of micro-organisms. By maintaining a stable and favourable gut flora it is possible to prevent pathogen colonization. This forms the basis for use of so-called 'probiotic' products, which are single or mixed cultures of 'beneficial' bacteria which complement energy and vitamin production, or bind to the same sites on the gut wall as pathogenic species, thereby reducing the ability for a pathogen to multiply to disease levels.

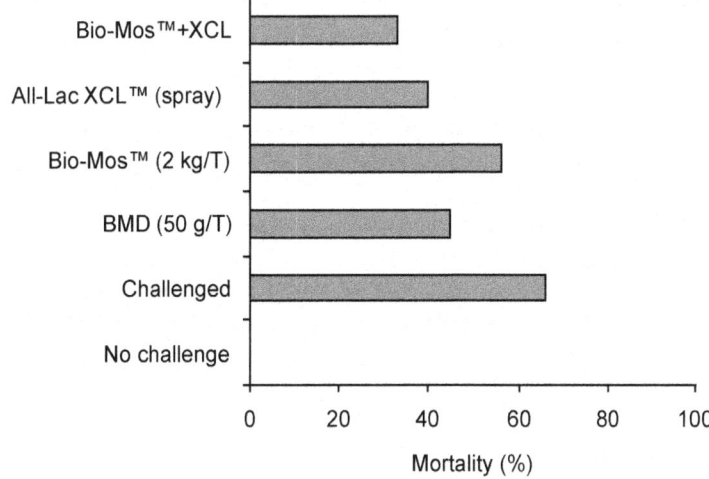

Figure 3.
Effects of different supplementation strategies on mortality in nectoric enteritis challenge.

Enhancing resilience

The chemical release elicited by a disease challenge depresses production directly by influencing metabolism and indirectly by suppressing appetite and hence feed intake. While immune response is crucial to maintaining health the immune response itself depressed production.

The gut lining forms the interface between foreign, antigenic material (feed and flora) and the bird. Although most of these organisms are not pathogenic (do not cause disease directly) they do stimulate an immune response. An inappropriate immune response to gastrointestinal antigenic stimulation has a negative impact on feed efficiency, as it is energetically expensive and diverts nutrient utilisation away from growth. As with heat stress the fever response to foreign antigens depresses intake, which also reduces the energy available for production.

As oligosaccharides comprise a major communication method in the gut, certain oligosaccharides derived from the outer cell wall of specialist yeast strains have been shown to be useful in maintaining the gut environment. For example, the specialist mannan-oligosaccharide, Bio-Mos has the capacity to modulate the immune system and the gut microflora, bind a wide range of pathogens and preserve the integrity of the intestinal absorptive surface due to its useful carbohydrate-based structure.

Bio-Mos is capable of enhancing specific circulatory and secretory immunoglobulin synthesis in response to antigen exposure (Savage *et al* 1996). By improving both the extent and uniformity of the immune response Bio-Mos enhances flock health. Poorly immunized birds within the flock provide an opportunity for infectious disease to become established, significantly increasing the level of challenge to which the pen-mates are exposed. Vaccination failure and disease outbreaks are much more likely to occur in flocks with a non-uniform immune response. By improving the uniformity of the flock response to vaccination it is possible to significantly reduce the risk and consequence of exposure to infectious disease agents.

Fever is a part of any protective immune response. The negative impact that fever has on feed intake and hence animal performance is perceived as the cost of health insurance. The three-dimensional structure of the unique mannoprotein molecule in Bio-Mos enables it to suppress the fever response (Table 1).

Table 1.
Effect of Bio-Mos and AGP on body temperature in turkey poults after Salmonella challenge (Ferket, 2001).

Parameter	Control	Bio-Mos	Virginiamycin
Control	41.40	41.49	41.38
Challenge	41.80[a]	41.48[b]	41.73[a]
Change	+0.4 °C	N.C.	+0.35 °C

Means not sharing a letter differ significantly $P < 0.05$.

Decreasing feed passage

Vegetable protein sources such as soy, have a complicated cellular matrix structure and contain anti-nutritive factors that can limit or disrupt the digestion and absorption of nutrients. The cellular matrix consists of protein, starch, fibre, minerals, fats, and other nutrients intertwined in a very complex, and sometimes indigestible, structure, making it difficult for gut enzymes to effectively break down this matrix completely. Young animals with immature digestive systems, or animals with absorptive or digestive problems due to disease or bacterial challenge are even less efficient at utilising such ingredients.

Malasimilation for whatever reason increases nutrient through-flow to the caeca and consequently leads to destabilization of the caecal flora. Abnormally rapid multiplication of the proteolytic organisms like *Clostridium perfringens* causes pH changes that allow these potential pathogens to migrate up the small intestine. Further access to nutrients facilitates Clostridial blooms to occur in the small intestine and the toxins produced cause clinical necrotic enteritis.

Ensuring protein digestion via supplementation with effective protease feed enzymes complements feed processing and the endogenous enzymes of the digestive system to more completely break down this matrix, resulting in a more efficient and complete use of nutrients. Research shows that when animals are fed the protease Allzyme Vegpro, digestion and utilization of vegetable protein ingredients can be improved by 7%. This is more significant in animals with restricted digestive capabilities, be they young animals with immature digestive systems, or older animals that have been compromised by disease.
Evaluating the field data on alternatives

The EU ban on the use of many of the commonly used antibiotic pronutrients has created the opportunity for extensive evaluation of alternate programs. Unfortunately, most of the data generated during "on farm" testing is not available for public scrutiny and that which is reported is supply-company specific and is consequently viewed with scepticism. The plethora of potentially confounding factors present under field conditions make the data farm specific and in addition such trials seldom have a negative control thus making comparative analysis difficult. Field analysis does however remain an important step in the process of alternative program implementation.

Conclusions

The comprehensive multi-factorial model developed by Rosen provides a very effective means of comparing pronutrients. Extrapolation of research data to the field situation does however need special consideration.

The outcome of research conducted under controlled conditions may not accurately reflect commercial reality, and single studies provide no information on the impact of long-term pronutrient use. While the use of long-term field trials would adequately address these concerns, these studies are confounded and are often not sensitive enough to establish statistically significant differences between treatments.

Financial return remains the most important motivator for change and in a high-volume, low-margin business monetary benefit is frequently derived long before statistical significance. The Rosen model cannot take account of possible changes in end-product market value derived from the implementation of alternative production programme.

To be successful in terms of enhanced contribution alternative programs have to be designed to address the challenges specific to the 'on farm' situation.

References

Anderson, D.B., McCracken V.J., Aminov R.I., Simpson J.M., Mackie R.I., Verstegen M.W.A., and Gaskins H.R. (2000) Gut microbiology and growth-promoting antibiotics in swine. *Nutritional Abstracts and Reviews Series B: Livestock Feeds and Feeding.* **70**: 2: 101-108.

Avellaneda, G. E., Jingrang L., Tongrui L., M. D., Holfacre, C. L., and Maurer, J. J. (2003) *The impact of growth-promoting antibiotics on total poultry microbiota as well as enterococcus population present on poultry carcass.* Poultry Disease Research Center, University of Georgia. July 2003 Program and Abstracts, Congress of the World Veterinary Poultry Association.

Barnes, J.H. (2003) Clostridial Diseases, Chapter 23. 11th ed., in *Diseases of Poultry*: 23: 775.

Branton. S. L., Lott B. D., Deaton J. W., Moslin W. R., Austin F. W., Pote L. M., Keirs R. W., Latour M. A., and Day E. J.. (1997) The effect of added complex carbohydrates or added dietary fiber on necrotic enteritis lesions in broiler chickens. *Poultry Science.* **76**(1): 24-28.

Board R.G. and Fuller R. (1994) *Microbiology of the Avian Egg.* Chapman and Hall, London.

Chung, K.C. and Goeffert J.M. (1970) Growth of salmonella at low pH. *Journal of Food Science.* **35**: 326-328.

Collett, S.R. and Dawson K.A. (2001) Alternatives to subtherapeutic antibiotics: What are the options? How effective are they? *Poultry beyond 2005. 2nd International Poultry Broiler Nutritionist's Conference* Sheraton Rotorua, New Zealand.

Collett, S.R. (2003) The Value of Understanding Total Productivity. In: *Nutritional Biotechnology In The Feed and Food Industries.* Edited by Lyons, T.P. and Jacques, K.A. pp. 85-91. Nottingham University Press, Nottingham, UK.

Ferket, P.R. and M.A. Qureshi. (2001) *The Immune System in Poultry.* Department of Poultry Science, College of Agriculture and Life Sciences, North Carolina State University, Raleigh, NC 27695-7608.

Fernandez, F. (2001) Evaluation of the effect of mannan-oligosaccharides on the competitive exclusion of Salmonella Enteritidis colonization in broiler chicks. *Avian Pathology.*

29: 575-581

Hoerr, F. D. (2003) Mycotoxicoses. In: *Diseases of Poultry 11th edition*. pp 1103-1119.

Holfacre, C. L , Lee, M.D. and Maurer, J. (2003) Enhancing gut microflora and its effects of clostridium. *37th National Meeting on Poultry Health Processing*. Oct 9-11th, Ocean City, Maryland, pp. 106-108.

Hooge, D.M. (2003a) Broiler chicken performance may improve with MOS. *Feedstuffs* January 6, 2003: 11-13

Hooge, D.M. (2003b) Market turkey pen trials with dietary MOS. *Feedstuffs: in press*

Idris, Umelaalim, Lu, J. I., Lee, M.D., Sanchez, S.I., Hofacre, C.L., and Maurer, J.J. (2003) Factors affecting epidemiology of antibiotic-resistant campylobacter jejuni and campylobarcter coli. Program and abstracts, *Congress of the World Veterinary Poultry Association*.

Johnson, D. C. and C. Pinedo. (1971) Gizzard erosion and ulceration in Peru broilers. *Avian Diseases* **15**: 835-837.

Kaldhusdal, M. and Skjerve, E. (1996) Association between cereal contents in the diet and incidence of necrotic enteritis in broiler chickens in Norway. *Preventative Veterinary Medicine* **28**: 1-16.

Kaldhusdal, M. and Hofshangen M. (1997) Barley inclusion and avoparcin supplementation in broilder diets. 2. Clincial, pathological and bacteriological findings in a mild form of necrotic enteritis. *Poultry Science* **71**: 1145-1153.

Kenyon, S. (2003) Personal communication

Klasing, K.C. (1998) Nutritional modulation of resistance to infectious diseases. *Poultry Science.* **77**: 1119-1125.

Lilijebjelke, K. A., and Hofacre, C., Liu T. and Maurer, J. (2003) Molecular epidemiology of salmonella on poultry farms in NE Georgia. Program and Abstracts, *Congress of the World Veterinary Poultry Association*.

Lukert, P.D. and Saif Y.M. (1995) Infectious Bursal Disease, in *Diseases of Poultry* (11th edition) chapter 6 pp161-173.

Martinez, R. and Wobeser G. (1999) Immunization of ducks for type C botulism. *Journal of Wildlife Diseases* **35**: 710-715.

Partanen, K. (2001) Organic acids - Their efficacy and modes of action. In: *Gut Environment of Pigs* Edited by Piva, A., Bach Knudsen, K.E. and Lindberg, J.E. pp. 79-96. Nottingham University Press, Nottingham, UK.

Partanen, K.H. and Mroz, Z. (1999) *Nutrition Research Reviews.* **12**: 117-145.

Rosen G. D. (2003) Setting and meeting standards for the efficient replacement of pronetrient antibiotics in broiler, turkey and pig nutrition. Personal communication

Rosen, G.D. (2000b) Enzymes for broilers: A multi-factorial assessment. *Feed International* **21**(12): 14-18.

Rosen, G.D. (2000a) Multi-factorial assessment of exogenous enzymes in broiler pronutrition: Target and problems. In: *Proceedings of the 3rd European Symposium on Feed Enzymes, Noordwijkerhout, Netherlands, 8-10 May, 2000:* in press

Rosen, G.D. (2001) Multi-factorial efficacy evaluation of alternatives to antimicrobials in pronutrition. *British Poultry Science* **42(S1):** S104-S105.

Rosen, G.D. (1995) Antibacterials in poultry and pig nutrition. In: *Biotechnology in the Animal Feeds and Animal Feeding* Edited by Wallace R.J. and Chesson A. pp. 143-172. VCH Verlagsgesellschaft, Weinheim, Germany.

Rosen, G.D. (1996) Feed additive nomenclature. *World Poultry Science Journal*. **52**: 53-57.

Rosen, G.D. (1996) *Proceedings of the World's Poultry Science Society*, Vol. II, p141. New Delhi.

Rosen, G.D. (198) Biotic nomeclature revisited. Letter to the editor *World Poultry Science Journal*. **54**: 99.

Schat, K.A. (2003) Circovirus Infections. In: *Diseases of Poultry, 11th edition.* pp 181-209.

Schildknect, E.; L. Rakebrand, L. Jensen, and Skinner*. (2003a) *Changes in live performance of broiler chickens raised on built-up litter for eight production cycles following a coccidiosis.* Alpharma Inc., Fort Lee, NJ. January 2003 International Poultry Scientific Forum Abstracts. **35**: 9.

Schildknect, E.; L. Rakebrand, L. J. and Skinner. (2003b) *Changes In Anticoccidial Sensitivity Profiles Of Coccidia From Broiler Chickens Raised On Built-Up Litter For Eight Production Cycles Following A Coccidiosis Challenge.* Alpharma Inc., Fort Lee, NJ January 2003 International Poultry Scientific Forum Abstracts. **36**: 10.

Siegel H.S. (1994) Stress and Immunity In *Proc 9th European Poultry Conference* Glasgow UK pp 122-125

Ten Doeschate, R.A.H.M. and Kenyon, S. (1999) Alternatives to antibiotic growth promoters: Mannan oligosaccharides and organic acids. In: *Proceedings of XIV European Symposium on the quality of poultry meat, Bologna, Italy*. Ed. Cavalchini, L.G. and Baroli, D.

Vaughan, E. E., Schut, F., Heilig, H.G.H.J., Zoetendal, E.G., de Vos, W.M. and Akkermans, A.D.L. (2000) A molecular view of the intestinal ecosystem. *Current Issues In Intestinal Microbiology*. **1**:(1): 1-12

Wages D. P., *Managing Poultry without Antibiotics*. (2003) 37th National Meeting On Poultry Health A Processing. Oct 9-11th, Ocean City, Maryland. pp 102-105.

Wages, D.P. and Opengart K. (2003a) Gangrenous Dermatitis. In: *Diseases of Poultry, 11th edition*. pp 791-794.

Wages, D.P. and Opengart K. (2003b) Necrotic Enteritis. In: *Diseases of Poultry, 11th edition.* pp 781-783.

Wang, R., Li, D., and Bourne, S. (1998) Can 2000 years of herbal medicine history help us solve problems in the year 2000? In: *Biotechnology in the Feed Industry.* Edited by T.P. Lyons and K.A. Jacques. Nottingham University Press, Nottinghams. Nottingham University Press, Nottingham pp. 273-291.

Witter, R. L. and Schat K. A. (1997) Marek's Disease. In: *Diseases of Poultry, 11th edition.* pp 407-446.

Wobeser, G. (1997) Avian botulism – another perspective. *Journal of Wildlife Diseases* **33**: 181-186.

Impact of mannan oligosaccharide on gut health and pig performance

Peter Spring

Swiss College of Agriculture, CH-3052 Zollikofen, Switzerland

Introduction

A healthy digestive system is crucial for optimal animal performance. However, the gut with it's large surface area and heavy microbial load, is a vulnerable site for pathogen entry into the body. This large surface is necessary to optimise nutrient absorption. To allow an efficient transfer of nutrients to the blood, the gut is protected with only one layer of epithelial cells. Unfortunately however, this thin layer does not only facilitate nutrient transfer, but also weakens the ability of the gastro intestinal (GI) tract to prevent pathogens from entering the body.

Therefore, a multitude of additional protection systems exist to minimise the risk of intestinal disease and pathogen entry. Mucins and glycoproteins associated with the intestinal brush border serve as important barriers protecting the delicate absorptive surface from the abrasive action of feedstuffs, bacterial colonisation, and toxins. Endogenous acids, digestive enzymes and bile reduce bacterial growth. Digestive flow and peristaltic movements transport the digesta through the digestive tract, and with it bacteria, thus limiting bacterial attachment and subsequent development. To further optimise gut protection the animal has devoted more than half of its immune cells to protecting the digestive tract. In addition, the GI microflora plays a crucial role in gut defence; through different complex mechanisms beneficial bacteria limit the growth of pathogens, trying to exclude them from the system (Rolfe, 1991).

Profound knowledge of the development and composition of the GI microflora and its regulatory forces is essential to understand the dynamics of the GI microflora as well as interactions with feedstuffs and feed additives.

93

Competitive exclusion

Competitive exclusion (CE) implies the prevention of entry or establishment of one bacterial population into the GI tract because a competing bacterial population already occupies that. To be able to succeed, the latter population must be better suited to establish or maintain itself in that environment or must produce compounds inhibitory to its competition (Bailey, 1987). Nurmi and Rantala (1973) were the first to apply the CE concept to domestic animals more than 30 years ago. The mechanisms, which are involved in CE, are very complex, since bacterial populations have a variety of different approaches to out-compete invaders (Table1).

Table 1.
Indirect and direct bacterial regulatory mechanisms which affect the composition of the microbial flora in the GI tract [a].

Regulatory mechanism	Control factors
Indirect mechanism:	
Induction of immunological process	- Intestinal Ig
Modification of bile salts	- Unconjugated bile acids
Influencing mucus production	- Mucus
Stimulation of peristalsis	- Flow rate
Direct mechanism:	
Nutrient utilisation	- Competition for nutrients or growth factors
	- Synergistic nutrient utilisation
Attachment	- Competition for receptor sites
	- Stimulation of epithelial cell turnover
Creation of a restrictive environment	- pH
	- Lactic acid
	- VFA
	- Hydrogen sulfide
	- Eh
	- Modification of bile salts
	- Induction of immunologic process
Production of antimicrobial substances	- Ammonia
	- Hydrogen peroxide
	- Hemolysin
	- Bacterial enzymes
	- Bacteriophage
	- Bacteriocins
	- Antibiotics

[a] Adapted from Miles (1993), Rolfe (1991) and Savage (1987)

These approaches can be divided into direct and indirect mechanisms. Indirect mechanisms are the result of the normal microbial flora altering the physiologic response of the host, which in turn affects the interaction between the host and micro-organism (Rolfe, 1991). Direct mechanisms are exerted by different bacterial populations upon each other. The complexity of the interactions makes it extremely difficult to study the effects of one isolated factor; we still do not understand most mechanisms involved in CE in detail nor do we know the exact function that each bacterial population plays in the gut. However, through nutrition we have the potential to influence any of the control mechanisms.

Two basic nutritional approaches can be applied to promote the beneficial GI microflora. First, by feeding beneficial bacteria (probiotics) we can support and complement the endogenous microflora. The effect of probiotics is well documented in the literature. For example, Hollister et al. (1999) reduced salmonella colonisation in chicks by feeding a live caecal culture from salmonella-free poultry. Fedorka-Cray et al. (1999) have shown a similar response to microbial cultures in young pigs. Gram-positive bacteria, including Lactobacillus, Enterococcus, Pediococcus, Bacillus, and Bifidobacteria, and fungi of the Saccharomyces (yeast) genus are often fed after antibiotic therapy as a means of re-introducing a beneficial flora to the gut of affected animals.

A second possibility to influence the outcome of bacterial competition comes through supporting certain specific mechanisms, which have an impact on CE. This can be achieved by modifying the composition of the diet or through the use of feed additives.

One of the key parameters influencing CE is the intestinal environment, particularly intestinal acid concentrations and pH. Beneficial bacteria inhibit the colonisation of pathogens by producing volatile fatty and lactic acids that reduce the pH in the digesta and of the brush-border microenvironment. Organic acids have strong antibacterial effects, especially to gram-negative pathogens. Mathew et al. (1996) demonstrated that during the weaning phase of the piglet, this mechanism is weakened and as a result the piglet is particularly susceptible to digestive upsets and diarrhoea. Figure 1 shows how some of the dietary factors can interfere with mechanisms involved in CE. The gut environment can be optimised by controlling buffering capacity and through addition of dietary acids. This approach has proven very effective in piglets since support is provided specifically in an area where the native protection is weakened.

Enhancing the digestibility of the diet leaves little substrate for bacterial fermentation and therefore stiffens bacterial competition for nutrients. This can be achieved by selecting highly digestible ingredients or by enhancing diet digestibility with thermal treatments or enzyme addition.

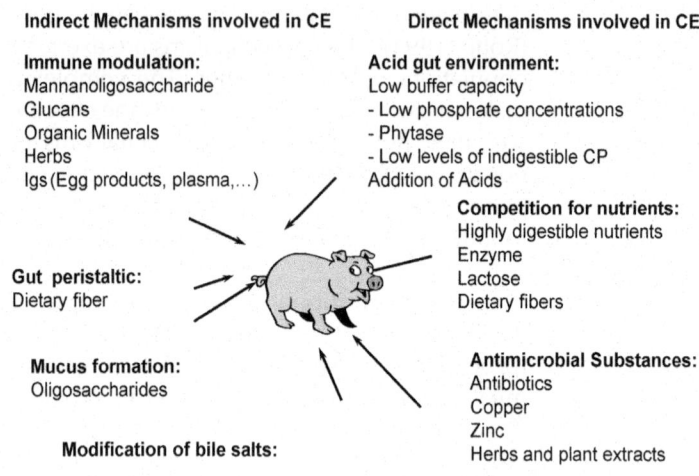

Indirect Mechanisms involved in CE   Direct Mechanisms involved in CE

Immune modulation:
Mannanoligosaccharide
Glucans
Organic Minerals
Herbs
Igs (Egg products, plasma,...)

Acid gut environment:
Low buffer capacity
- Low phosphate concentrations
- Phytase
- Low levels of indigestible CP
Addition of Acids

Competition for nutrients:
Highly digestible nutrients
Enzyme
Lactose
Dietary fibers

Gut peristaltic:
Dietary fiber

Mucus formation:
Oligosaccharides

Antimicrobial Substances:
Antibiotics
Copper
Zinc
Herbs and plant extracts

Modification of bile salts:

Attachment:
Mannan oligosaccharide

Figure 1. Strengthening the beneficial bacteria and inhibiting pathogens by supporting mechanisms involved in competitive exclusion.

The antimicrobial metabolites produced by the native gut micro-organism include a wide range of inhibitory substances. Lactobacilli have been extensively studied for production of antagonists. Several antibiotic-like substances with activity against Gram-positive and Gram-negative bacteria have been isolated (Gilliland, 1989). Reuterin, for example, is produced by *Lactobacillus reuteri* under anaerobic conditions at a pH and temperature similar to those in the small intestine of animals (Juven *et al.*, 1991). Through nutrition we can mimic these mechanisms by adding natural antimicrobial compounds such as essential oils from oregano which contains phenolic compounds, such as carvacrol, that have antimicrobial properties (Akagul and Kivanc, 1988).

Blomberg *et al.* (1993) also demonstrated that undefined compounds in a culture of lactobacilli inhibit the attachment of pathogenic *E. coli* K88 to intestinal components of pigs. They suggested that compounds produced by the lactobacilli or the lactobacilli themselves are binding to the receptor of *E. coli* K88, thereby preventing its colonisation. Research by Oyofo and co-worker (1989a; b; c) suggests that mannan-type sugars play a role in bacterial attachment.

The gut is a major interface where the immune system can sample potential antigens in the animal's environment and if necessary mount a defensive strategy to resist disease. Therefore, the resident microflora will have a marked effect on the amount and profile of immune factors, such as immunoglobulins (Ig). Perdigon *et al.* (1991)

observed that specific lactobacilli fed to mice resulted in enhanced protection against *Salmonella typhimurium* and *E. coli* by increasing IgA production. The diet can interact with the immune system in the same way as the microflora. Certain dietary ingredients can modulate gut-associated humoral immunity and immunoglobulins can also be added directly to the diet. For example, to produce specific antibodies, laying hens are exposed to particular antigens to stimulate the production of immunoglobulins, which are then deposited in the egg. These immunoglobulins are subsequently harvested from the eggs and fed to susceptible young animals. Plasma protein can be used as a source of non-specific antibodies, where feeding animal protein is still allowed by the regulatory body.

Nutrition offers an array of possibilities to influence the natural mechanisms, which are involved in CE. Field experience suggests that different approaches should be taken simultaneously in order to maximise gut health. An ingredient that is extensively used in the field to enhance gut health is mannan oligosaccharide (MOS) derived from yeast. Research suggests that MOS interferes with bacterial attachment and can also interact with the immune system. As MOS is a non-viable product it does not classify as a CE culture. It could rather be classified as a prebiotic or more general as an intestinal microflora modulator.

Interactions of mannan oligosaccharide with the GI microflora

The initial interest in using mannan oligosaccharide (MOS; Bio-Mos® Alltech Inc.) for pathogen adsorption originated from work performed in the late 1980s investigating the ability of mannose to inhibit salmonella infection in broilers. Oyofo *et al.* (1989a; b; c) demonstrated inhibition of adherence of *Salmonella typhimurium* to the epithelial cells from the GI tract of 1-d-old chicks in the presence of mannose *in vitro*. They also showed a reduction in the caecal concentration of *S. typhimurium* with dietary mannose in broilers. Similar results have been demonstrated with MOS at significantly lower concentrations than that required for purified mannose (Spring, 1996). Studies have been conducted to compare the ability of different mannose-type sugars to block bacterial attachment by pathogenic bacteria expressing type 1 fimbriae to D-mannose. D-mannose-6-phosphate or ß-bonded 1, 4 mannan do not bind *E. coli* to any appreciable degree. In contrast, mannan molecules bound in α-1, 3 linkages demonstrate slightly higher binding capacity than pure D-mannose. For example, Firon *et al.* (1983) demonstrated that a compound containing both α-1, 3 and α-1, 6 branched mannans had approximately 37.5 times the binding capacity for *E. coli* as D-mannose. A number of references show that the side chains of certain strains of *Saccharomyces cerevisiae* end in an α-1, 3 linked end unit to an α-1, 6 backbone mannan structure with varying concentrations of α-1, 2 linked end units (Ballou, 1976; Cabib and Roberts, 1982). This relatively greater functional binding capacity and the resistance of MOS to digestion might help to explain why changes in the gut microflora have been observed with MOS at lower inclusion levels compared with mannose. The variation among strains of *S. cerevisiae* in the chemical configuration of the cell wall should be examined when selecting a suitable strain for agglutination of pathogenic bacteria.

In preliminary University animal trials, MOS was shown to reduce the prevalence and concentration of different strains of salmonella as well as *E. coli* in the caecum of broiler chicks challenged with those strains of bacteria. (Figure 2; Spring *et al.*, 2000).

Figure 2. Effect of dietary MOS on cecal *E. coli* 15r concentrations of chicks maintained in microbial isolators (p < 0.05).

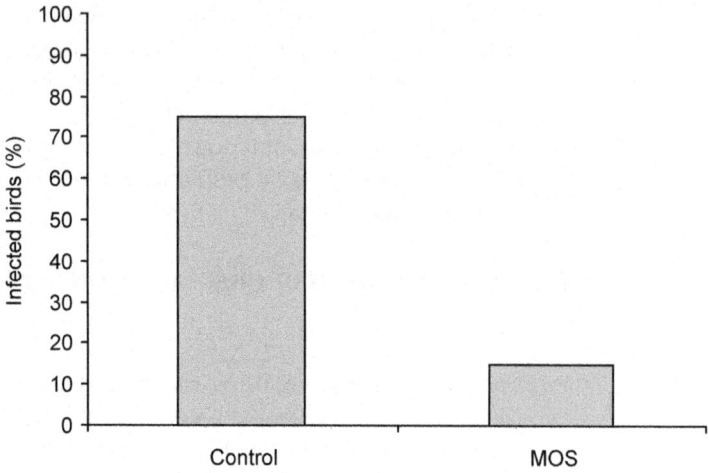

These preliminary findings have also been confirmed under field conditions. Mannan oligosaccharide has been shown to reduce salmonella colonisation in the caecum as well as in the liver and spleen in naturally challenged broiler flocks (Figure 3) and to reduce faecal *E. coli* concentrations in piglets and calves.

In a recent piglet trial, a reduction in *Clostridium perfringens* was reported with dietary MOS (Figure 4). Clostridia are not known to express type-1-fimbriae and therefore would not be expected to undergo agglutination by MOS. However, it might be possible that MOS brings about the reduction by improving overall gut health or by its effect on the immune response.

Different studies have investigated the interaction of MOS with the immune system and have reported enhanced macrophage activity

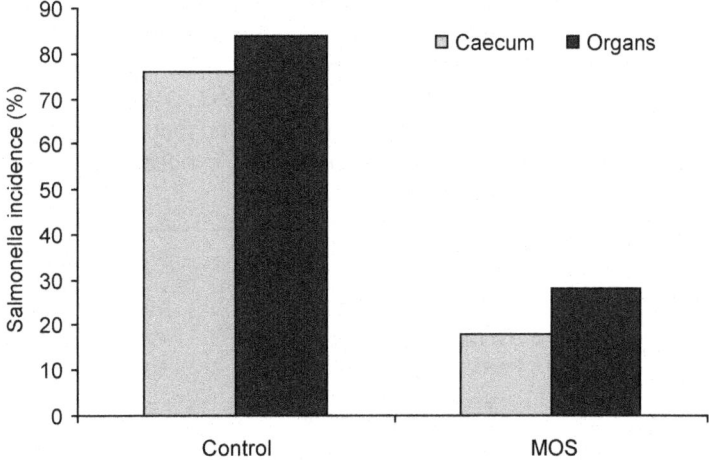

Figure 3.
Effect of MOS
on Salmonella
prevalence in
broiler chicks
(Sisak, 1994).

and humoral immunity. There is also some evidence that MOS may down regulate the pro-inflammatory immune response that is detrimental to growth and production (Ferket, 2002). Under commercial conditions where animals are subjected to chronic immunological stress, MOS could enhance appetite by reducing the pro-inflammatory immune response.

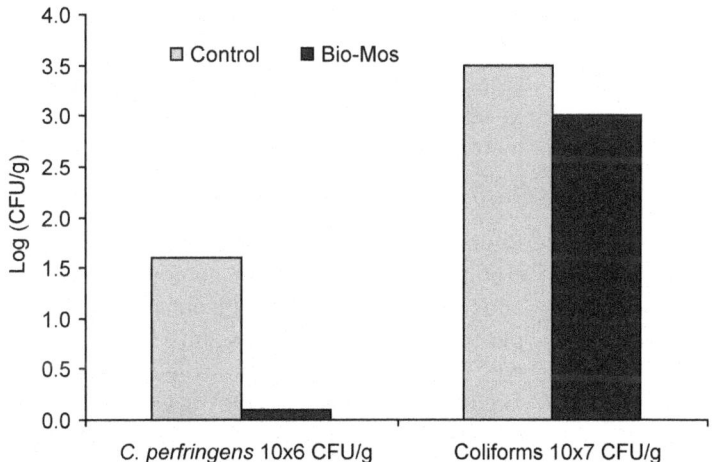

Figure 4.
Effect of MOS
on Clostridia in
piglets (personal
communication,
Geliot).

Effects of MOS on piglet performance

The restriction on using antibiotic growth promoters challenges the pig producer to improve management in order to minimise gastrointestinal dysfunction and mortality in piglets. Despite significant efforts in this direction, many producers have experienced more piglet diarrhoea post-weaning. A large dataset is available on the effect of MOS (Bio-Mos®) on piglet health and performance, with a recent meta-analysis of 49 comparisons (Table 2) showing an average improvement in weight gain of more than 4% and feed conversion ratio of 2-3% (Miguel and Pettigrew, 2002). In particular, the results showed that performance responses appeared larger where animals were exposed to stressors and were therefore performing sub-optimally.

Table 2. Growth rate, feed intake and feed/gain response to Bio-Mos® in starting pigs.

Parameter	n	% Difference[1]	SEM
Average daily gain	49	+ 4.18	0.77*
Average daily feed intake	49	+ 2.14	0.67*
Feed conversion ratio	49	- 2.24	0.51*

[1] Bio-Mos® - control, % of control
*$P < 0.05$

MOS is applied in a step down program to ensure sufficient MOS is consumed, especially in very young piglets with low feed intakes. The recommended inclusions are 4kg/t in pre-starter diets, plus 2kg/t and 1kg/t in the starter-1 and starter-2 diets, respectively. Evidence to date indicates this is an effective strategy.

Effects of MOS on sow performance

Until recently, little information has been available on the potential to improve piglet immunity by feeding MOS to sows, thereby increasing colostrum quality as a side effect of boosting the sow's own immune system.

Preliminary data generated under University conditions where confirmed in a large-scale commercial trial involving 1,016 sows and 10,127 piglets carried out in North Carolina in 2001. Sow performance on the unit's standard commercial diets was compared with that of sows fed the same diets reformulated to include 2kg/t and 1kg/t of MOS (Bio-Mos®) during gestation and lactation, respectively (by substituting MOS for an equivalent weight of corn). These inclusion levels were designed to supply approximately 5g MOS/sow/day (O'Quinn et al., 2001).

Five hundred and nine sows were transferred onto the treatment diets at 21 days pre-farrowing, through until the end of lactation (21 days post-farrowing). Significant improvements were observed in average birth weight and daily liveweight gain ($p < 0.05$ and $p < 0.01$, respectively) where sows were fed MOS, though the results (Table 3) show no differences in sow weights, number of pigs born alive or stillborns. MOS-supplementation resulted in a superior weaning weight (5.47 kg compared to 5.80 kg, (P < 0.01), with pre-weaning mortality falling to just 9.09% (P < 0.01). Adjusted for equal weaning age the weight difference would be close to 400 grams extra weight at weaning.

Table 3.
Large-scale commercial evaluation of MOS in sow diets (O'Quinn et al., 2001).

		Treatment		
		Control	MOS*	p
Sows per treatment (no.)		517	509	
Parity (no.)		3.23	3.29	n.s.
MOS dose rate (kg/t):	Gestation	0.0	2.0	
	Lactation	0.0	1.0	
Initial sow weight (kg)		263.5	265.3	n.s.
Final sow weight (kg)		235.7	236.9	n.s.
Piglets alive at processing [†] (no.)		9.96	9.78	n.s.
Stillborn (no.)		1.06	1.05	n.s.
Lactation length (days)		21.10	20.76	< 0.05
Return to oestrus (days)		7.27	5.20	< 0.01
Pre-weaning mortality (%)		11.27	9.09	< 0.01
Average birth weight (kg)		1.66	1.70	< 0.05
Average weaning weight (kg)		5.47	5.80	< 0.01
Daily liveweight gain (g/d)		177	195	< 0.01
Total weight gain (kg)		3.80	4.12	< 0.01

Note: [*] Supplied in the form of Bio-Mos; [†] approx. 30 hours post-farrowing

One of the more intriguing results from this particular trial was the substantial reduction in the time taken for sows to return to oestrus, cut by 2.07 days with MOS addition. This response was significant (P < 0.01), although there is no clear explanation and no measurements were taken to determine any potential mode of action. However, it is suggested that any enhancement in immune status would speed recovery from sub-clinical infections picked up during farrowing, with consequent benefits for fertility.

The trial also reported a significant increase in the concentrations of certain immunoglobulins (antibodies) found in the colostrum from the sows fed MOS (Table 4). In particular, significant improvements were found in both Immunoglobulin G (Ig G) and Immunoglobulin M (Ig M) concentrations, along with a strong trend towards improved Immunoglobulin A (Ig A) levels.

Table 4.
Effect of MOS on colostrum immunoglobulin concentrations (O'Quinn, et al., 2001)

Parameter	Colostrum immunoglobulin concentration (mg/dL)		
	Control	MOS*	p
Immunoglobulin A	1,097	1,178	0.06
Immunoglobulin G	4,842	5,853	0.007
Immunoglobulin M	241	273	0.03

Note: [*] Supplied in the form of Bio-Mos®.

The performance results are supported by a series of follow up trials involving 2500 sows conducted in University herds and commercial units in the US, Italy, Croatia and Spain. Overall analyses reveal a significant improvement in weaning weight (Figure 5) and a significant (P < 0.01) reduction in pre-weaning mortality with MOS (11.47 % vs. 9.71%).

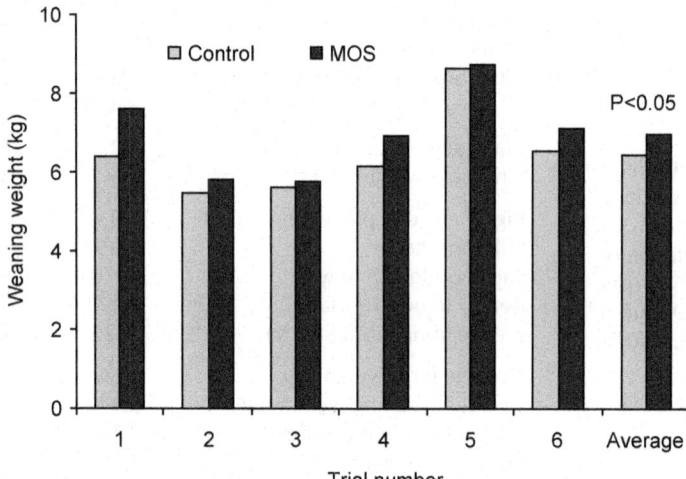

Figure 5.
Effect of MOS fed to the sow on weaning weight of piglets (adapted from Spring and Geliot, 2003).

Colostrum represents the accumulated secreted antibodies of the mammary gland. In pigs the placenta is epithelichorial, which means that the fetal chorionic epithelium is in contact with intact uterine epithelium. In this type of placentation, transplacental passage of immunoglobulins is prevented making the newborn piglet entirely dependent on antibodies present in the colostrum. It is clear that improvements in colostrum quality can have a crucial impact on performance. It is widely recognised, for example, that IgA plays an important function in gut protection during the first days of a piglet's life, and any improvement in colostrum levels is clearly desirable. Researchers are also examining the potential role of EGFs (Epithelial growth factors) in colostrum and milk from MOS fed sows. The combination of improved immune status, plus the reduction in microbial contamination of the farrowing crate through direct MOS effects on the sow, may improve the intestinal microbial population of the piglet and with it reduce infections and diarrhoea. Maxwell *et al.* (2003) reported reduced incidence of piglet diarrhoea with MOS-supplementation of sow diets. Whatever the true mechanism, the opportunity to protect growth rates at such an early age without the blanket use of antibiotics is clearly of benefit to all those involved in modern pig production. With pressure to adopt more consumer-friendly practices continuing to increase, the use of natural additives in the sow's feed to provide that protection is clearly a step forwards.

Conclusions

- The beneficial microflora plays a key role in controlling intestinal pathogens.

- Nutrition offers an array of possibilities to influence the GI microflora and thus improving gut health.

- Mannan oligosaccharide reduces intestinal pathogens through pathogen binding and by improving the immune defence. Therefore, its use has a role in food safety.

- MOS has been shown to improve piglet performance when being added to either the piglet and/or sow diets.

References

Akagul, A., and Kivanc, M. (1988) Inhibitory effects of selected Turkish spices and oregano compounds on some food-borne fungi. *International Journal of Food Microbiology* **6**: 264-268.

Bailey, J.S. (1987) Factors affecting microbial competitive exclusion in poultry. *Food Technology* **41**: 88-92.

Ballou, C. (1976) Structure and biosynthesis of the mannan component of the yeast cell envelope. In: *Advances In Microbiological Physiology*. Edited by. Rose and Tempest Vol. 11, pp. 93-158.

Blomberg, L.A., Henriksson, and Conway, P.L. (1993) Inhibition of adhesion of *Escherichia coli* K88 to piglet ileal mucus by *Lactobacillus spp. Applied Environmental Microbiology* **59**: 34-39.

Cabib, E. and Roberts, R. (1982) Synthesis of the yeast cell wall and its regulation. *Annual Review of Biochemistry* **51**: 763-793.

Fedorka-Cray, P.J., Bailey, J.S., Stern, N.J., Cox, N.A., Ladely, S.R., and Musgrove, M. (1999) Mucosal competitive exclusion to reduce Salmonella in swine. *Journal of Food Protection* **62**:1376-1380.

Ferket, P.R. (2002) Use of oligosaccharides and gut modifiers as replacements for dietary antibiotics. *Proceedings of the 63rd Minnesota Nutrition Conference*, September 17-18, Eagan, MN, pp. 169-182.

Finucane, M.C., Dawson K.A., Spring P., and Newman, K.E. (1999) The effect of mannan oligosaccharide on the composition of the microflora in turkey poults. *Poultry Science* **78**(Suppl. 1): 77.

Firon, N., Ofek, I., and Sharon, N. (1983) Carbohydrate specificity of the surface lectins of *Escherichia coli, Klebsiella pneumoniae* and *Salmonella typhimurium. Carbohydrate Research* **120**: 235-249.

Gilliland, S.E. (1989) Acidophilus milk products: A review of potential benefits to customers. *Journal of Dairy Science* **72**: 2483-2494.

Hollister, A.G., Corrier, D.E., Nisbet, D.J., and DeLoach, J.R. (1999) Effects of chicken-derived cecal microorganisms maintained in continuous culture on cecal colonization by *Salmonella typhimurium* in turkey poults. *Poultry Science* **78**: 546-549.

Juven, B.J., Meinersmann, R.J., and Stern, M.J. (1991) Antagonistic effects of lactobacilli and pediococci to control intestinal colonization by human enteropathogens in live poultry. *Journal of Applied Bacteriology* **70**: 95-103.

Mathew, A.G., Franklin M.A., Upchruch, W.G., and Chattin, S.E. (1996) Influence of waning age on ileal microflora and fermentation acids in young pigs. *Nutrition Research* **16**: 817-827.

Maxwell, C. V., Ferrell, K., Dvorak, R. A., Johnson, Z. B., and Davis, M.E. (2003) Efficacy of mannan oligosaccharide supplementation through late gestation and lactation on sow and litter performance. *Journal of Animal Science* **81** (Suppl. 2): 69.

Miguel, J.C., Rodrigues-Zas, S.L., and Pettigrew, J.E. (2002) Practical effects of Bio-Mos in nursery pig diets: a meta-analysis. In: *Nutritional Biotechnology in the Feed and Food Industry.* Edited by Lyons T.P. and Jacques K.A. pp. 425-434. Nottingham University Press, Nottingham, UK.

Miles, R.D. (1993) Manipulation of the microflora of the gastrointestinal tract. Natural ways to prevent colonization by pathogens. In: *Biotechnology in the Feed Industry* Edited by Lyons, T.P. pp. 133-50. Nottingham University Press, Nottingham, UK.

Newman, K.E., and Newman, M.C. (2001) Evaluation of Bio-Mos (mannan-oligosaccharide) on the microflora and immunoglobulin status of sows: Part 1. Sow immunoglobulin status and piglet performance. *Journal of Animal Science* **79**(Suppl. 1): 189.

Nurmi, E., and Rantala, M.W. (1973) New aspect of salmonella infection in broiler production. *Nature* **241**: 210-211.

O'Quinn, P.R., Funderburke, D.W., and Tibbetts, G.W. (2001) Effects of dietary supplementation with mannan oligosaccharides on sow and litter performance in commercial production systems. *Journal of Animal Science* **79**(Suppl. 1): 212.

Oyofo, A.O., DeLoach, J.R., Corrier, D.E., Norman, J.O., Ziprin, R.L., and Mollenhauer, H.H. (1989a) Effect of carbohydrates on *Salmonella typhimurium* colonization in broiler chickens. *Avian Disease* **33**: 531-534.

Oyofo, A.O., DeLoach, J.R., Corrier ,D.E., Norman, J.O., Ziprin, R.L., and Mollenhauer, H.H. (1989b) Prevention of *Salmonella typhimurium* colonization of broilers with D-mannose. *Poultry Science* **68**: 1357-1360.

Oyofo, B.A., Droleskey, R.E., Norman, J.O., Mollenhauer, H.M., Ziprin, R.L., Corrier, D.E. and Deloach, J.R. (1989c) Inhibition by mannose of *in vitro* colonization of chicken small intestine by *Salmonella typhimurium*. *Poultry Science* **68**: 1351-1356.

Perdigon, G., Alvarez, S., and Pesce deRuiz Holdago, A. (1991) Immuno-adjuvant activity of oral *Lactobacillus casei*: influence of dose on the secretory immune response and protective capacity in intestinal infections. *Journal of Dairy Research* **58**: 485-496.

Rolfe, R.D. (1991) Population dynamics of the intestinal tract. In: *Colonization control of human enteropathogens in poultry* Edited by Blankenship L.C. pp. 59-75. Academic Press, Inc., San Diego, CA.

Savage, D.C. (1987) Factors influencing bio-control of bacterial pathogens in the intestine. *Food Technology* **41**: 82-87.

Sisak, F. (1994) Stimulation of phagocytosis as assessed by luminal-enhanced chemiluminescence and response to salmonella challenge of poultry fed diets containing mannan oligosaccharides. Abstract presented at Alltech's 10th Annual Symposium on Biotechnology in the Feed Industry, May 1994, Lexington, Kentucky.

Spring, P. (1996) *Effect of mannanoligosaccharide on different cecal parameters and on cecal concentration of enteric pathogens in poultry*. Dissertation. Federal Institute of Technology, Zurich, Switzerland.

Spring, P., and Geliot, P. (2003) Effetto di diete contenenti mannanoligosaccaridi sulle prestazioni delle scrofe. *Meeting Annuale della SIPAS*, Salsomaggiore, Italy. March 27th and 28th.

Spring, P., Wenk, C., Dawson, K.A., and Newman, K.E. (2000) The effects of dietary mannanoligosaccharides on cecal parameters and the concentrations of enteric bacteria in the ceca of salmonella-challenged broiler chicks. *Poultry Science* **79**: 205-211.

The potential for immunosaccharides to maximise growth performance – A review of six published meta-analyses on Bio-Mos

Andreas Kocher
Alltech Biotechnology Centre, Dunboyne, Ireland

Introduction

The role of indigestible oligo- and polysaccharides as substrates for the microflora in the large intestine of farm animals has been widely discussed in scientific literature. Additionally, it is well-known that the microflora plays a key role in the development of the gut-associated immune system (GALT) (Fioramonti *et al.* 2003). It has further been recognised that sugars on the intestinal surface have an important role in the bacterial attachment to the host (Firon *et al.* 1983; Ofek *et al.* 1977). However, it is only recently that carbohydrates have been recognised as being involved in almost every aspect of biology. Distinct carbohydrate structures can have very specific biological activities. For example, sugars (monosaccharides) combine to form giant molecules such as cellulose; they are already known to regulate hormones, organize embryonic development, direct the movement of cells and proteins throughout the body, and regulate the immune system (Schmidt 2002). Glycobiology or glycomics is defined as the characterisation of the sugars that make up a cell (Newman 2004). Understanding the structure and sequence of individual monosaccharides that form oligo- or polysaccharides is the base for developing new carbohydrate based immune-modulators. Research suggests that we can influence some of the control mechanisms of the immune system through selected dietary carbohydrates or immunosaccharides, as the digestive tract offers a large surface for carbohydrates to interact with intestinal cells and the immune system as well as with bacterial cells. It has been shown that the use of specific immunosaccharides (Bio-Mos®, Alltech Inc.) have a profound effect on animal health and subsequently animal performance. Advantages of adding Bio-Mos® to broiler, turkey, pig and rabbit diets have been evaluated in six individual meta-analyses and have recently been published in scientific journals and trade magazines.

107

Nutrition and immunity

The development of a rapid immune response is a key element in maximising animal growth performance. A variety of antigens in the environment, bacteria, viruses, protozoa, fungi and other parasites can have a significant impact on animal health, and subsequently on growth performance and reproduction. The reason for reduced productivity is not only the pathological consequence of the antigen, but also a direct consequence of the immune response of the host. It has been estimated that the demand for specific nutrients such as lysine and trace minerals for the production of lymphocytes and the synthesis of immunoglobulins during an immune response will increase by 5% and 18% respectively (Klasing 2001). However, the biggest impact on nutrient availability and subsequent animal growth performance comes from the decrease in feed intake associated with the release of pro-inflammatory cytokines during the immune response, as well as the reduction in nutrient absorption due to immune response to pathogens (Koutsos and Klasing 2002). Preventing exposure to potential pathogens or other antigens that onset an acute immune response is the key for optimal animal growth performance. Modulation of both the innate (non-specific) and acquired (specific) immunity will increase the animal's ability to defend against a wide range of antigens. Innate immunity refers to naturally-occurring defence mechanisms such as phagocytic cells or inflammatory mediators, whereas the acquired immunity refers to the recognition of specific antigens. Enhancing the animal's ability to defend against potential antigens by increasing the level of antibody titres, immunoglobulins and macrophage activity indicates a greater capacity to cope with potential diseases and will ultimately lead to better health and better growth performance.

Tools to control exposure to antigens

The animal feed industry worldwide has historically been using antibiotics in farm animals at therapeutical levels to control actual disease and at subtherapeutical levels to promote growth and feed efficiency. The use of antimicrobial growth promoters (AGP) can reduce the exposure to bacterial antigens and therefore reduce the onset of an immune response. However, more recently, the use of antibiotics in animal feed has been widely debated. The main concerns are the loss of efficacy of AGPs and the emergence of antibiotic resistant human pathogens after the prolonged use of antibiotics in animal feed. As a result, many countries have already decided on the implementation of a ban of AGPs in all animal feed.

The challenge faced by animal producers is clearly to find alternate ways to prevent and manage disease in livestock production. New strategies to reduce the exposure to potential pathogens include strict biosecurity programs, the use of feed additives such as organic acids or probiotics and vaccination. Already, vaccines are widely used as an effective tool against specific diseases. Vaccines that enhance the production of specific immunoglobulins (humoral immune response) will minimise immunological stress and therefore have a positive impact on animal health with a minimal effect on growth performance. Vaccines are generally used to provoke a systemic immune response against a particular antigen. Furthermore, depending on the type of vaccine, vaccination could have a negative impact on growth performance due to the secretion of acute phase protein (Klasing 1998).

More recently the focus has shifted to nutritional strategies to modulate the immune system and resist disease. The gastrointestinal tract is the major interface between potential antigens and the immune system. In particular the microbial population in the intestine protects the host from the colonisation of potential pathogens as well as playing a major role in the development of the gut associated immune system (Moreau and Gaboriau-Routhiau, 2000). The interaction between the intestinal microflora, available nutrients and the immune system has a major influence on animal health and will ultimately determine animal growth performance.

The use of immunosaccharides to enhance immune function

Mannan oligosaccharides (for example, Bio-Mos® derived from the outer cell wall of a specific strain of *Saccharomyces cerevisiae* using a proprietary process developed by Alltech Inc.), have been shown to inhibit pathogen colonisation by blocking the type-1 fimbriae which enable these pathogens to attach to the intestinal lining. Blocking bacterial attachment sites can also lead to improved immunity by allowing pathogens to be presented to immune cells as attenuated antigens (Ferket, 2004). It is further suggested that Bio-Mos® has a direct effect on the immune cells in the gastrointestinal tract via its uptake into M-cells located in the Peyer's patches on the intestinal surface. The use of Bio-Mos® as an immunosaccharide has been demonstrated by Savage and Zakrzewska (1996) who reported that it increased plasma IgG and bile IgA in turkeys. In piglet diets it can lead to alteration in the leukocytes populations (Davis *et al.* 2004) and IgA titers in sow's milk (O'Quinn *et al.* 2001). Preventing the onset of an acute phase immune response with an immunosaccharide has a profound impact on growth performance.

Performance evaluation of dietary immunosaccharide

The evaluation of commercially available immunosaccharides is limited to one product only due to the fact that relevant animal performance data only exists for Bio-Mos®. To date, over 300 scientific trials on the use of immunosaccharides have been conducted to evaluate the potential benefits of Bio-Mos® on animal health and livestock performance. The advantages to broiler, turkey, pig and rabbit diets have been shown in six individual meta-analyses and have recently been published in scientific journals and trade magazines. The individual sets are based on published and unpublished data and include a total of 55 comparisons in nursery pigs (Pettigrew and Miguel, 2003), 5 comparisons in finishing pigs (Pettigrew, 2000), 44 comparisons in broilers (pen studies only) (Hooge, 2004a), 15 comparisons in broilers (field studies) (Hooge and Sefton, 2004), 27 comparisons in turkeys (Hooge, 2004b) and 20 comparisons in rabbits (Kocher et al., 2004). The effects of adding Bio-Mos® to diets were compared using the following parameters: bodyweight, feed conversion ratio (FCR) and mortality (for broilers, turkeys and rabbits); average daily gain, average daily feed intake and FCR (for pigs). Mean values of these parameters were analysed statistically as pairs of observations using a control vs. Bio-Mos® diet by the Paired T-test.

Pigs (Pettigrew, 2000; Pettigrew and Miguel, 2003)

The summary of the meta-analysis in nursing and finishing pigs is shown in Table 1. Inclusion levels varied between 1 –3 kg/t in nursery pigs and 0.5 – 2 kg/t for finishing pigs. Weaning weight had no significant effect on the performance response to Bio-Mos®.

Table 1. Response to Bio-Mos® in nursery and finishing pigs.

Nursery pigs	No. of comparisons	Difference (% of control)	p-value
Av. daily gain	55	4.15	0.001
Av. daily feed intake	55	2.08	0.001
FCR	55	-2.34%	0.001
Finishing pigs	No. of comparisons	Difference (% of control)	p-value
Av. daily gain	5	1.77	NS
Av. daily feed intake	5	5.41	NS
FCR	5	4.77	NS

The meta-analysis in nursery pigs demonstrated a 4.15% improved weight gain, 2.08% higher feed intake and a reduction in the feed conversion ratio by 2.34%. The improvements in all parameters are highly statistically significant and it can therefore clearly be stated that modulating the immune response by adding Bio-Mos® at 2 kg/t to nursery pig diets from weaning until 35 days of age has a significant impact on pig performance.

Due to the limited number of comparisons in finishing pigs it is difficult at this stage to obtain a clear picture on the possible benefits of Bio-Mos®. The data presented indicate improved growth performance in older pigs, however further research is necessary with finishing pigs.

Broilers (Hooge 2004a; Hooge and Sefton 2004)

The summary of the meta-analysis on the effects of Bio-Mos® in broilers diets is shown in Table 2. Due to the large number of pen trials it was possible to evaluate the effects compared with a negative control (no additive) as well as a positive control (AGP and coccidiostat). Furthermore a third meta-analysis was conducted evaluating the effects of Bio-Mos® in field trials under commercial conditions. All three comparisons show a significant improvement in liveability (reduction in mortality) when Bio-Mos® was added to the diet which clearly highlights a significant effect on the overall immune response in broilers and subsequent improvement in resistance to disease. An improvement in the overall health status of the birds is further highlighted by the improvement in FCR in all three comparisons. The improvement in FCR was significant when compared with a diet without any additive, and would indicate a profound effect on nutrient utilisation and bird health. In comparison with an unsupplemented diet, the addition of Bio-Mos® resulted in a significant improvement in weight gain. In comparison with an AGP control (pen studies and field studies) the addition of Bio-Mos® resulted in statistically similar body weight and numerically better (FCR) growth performance. Based on these results it can be stated that Bio-Mos® is a proven and economical feed additive for broiler diets. Currently recommended inclusion levels are: 2 kg/t in starter diet; 1 kg/t in grower diets and 0.5 kg/t in finisher and withdrawal diets.

Turkeys (Hooge, 2004b)

The summary of the meta-analysis on the effects of Bio-Mos® in turkey diets is presented in Table 3. No commercial field trials were included in this comparison. The typical inclusion levels followed a similar pattern as in broiler diets of 2 kg/t, 1kg/t and 0.5kg/t

Table 2. Response to Bio-Mos® in broilers diets

Pen trials	vs negative control			vs. AGP control		
	No. of comparisons	% difference	p-value	No. of comparisons	% difference	p-value
Body weight	44	+1.75%	0.001	26	-0.32%	NS
FCR	44	-1.89%	0.001	26	-0.44%	NS
Mortality	26	-16.4%	0.001	20	-17.2%	0.007

Field trials				vs mixed control*		
				No. of comparisons	% difference	p-value
Body weight				15	2.20	0.135
FCR				15	-2.02	0.025
Mortality				15	-24.1	0.004

* control incl. no additive, probiotics or AGP supplemented feed

Table 3. Response to Bio-Mos® in turkey diets

Pen trials	vs negative control			vs. AGP control		
	No. of comparisons	% difference	p-value	No. of comparisons	% difference	p-value
Body weight	27	+2.25%	0.006	20	-0.60%	NS
FCR	24	-1.55%	NS	20	-0.30%	NS
Mortality	16	-24.64%	0.05	15	-20.59%	0.07

Table 4. Response to Bio-Mos® in rabbit diets

Pen trials	vs negative control			vs. AGP control		
	No. of comparisons	% difference	p-value	No. of comparisons	% difference	p-value
Body weight	20	4.57%	0.001	9	-0.67%	NS
FCR	20	-5.08%	0.001	9	-1.87%	NS
Mortality	19	-49.04%	0.004	9	-28.72%	0.09

respectively. The inclusion of Bio-Mos® in turkey diets significantly improved body weight (+ 2.25%) and numerically improved FCR (-1.55%) compared with a negative control, whereas in comparison with an AGP control, the addition resulted in statistically similar growth performance. There was a very strong tendency (P < 0.07) to improve liveability of turkeys regardless of the control diet. In conclusion, Bio-Mos® can be considered an effective feed additive for improving live performance of turkeys.

Rabbits (Kocher *et al.* 2004)

In commercial rabbitries, enteric disorders after weaning are a continuing problem, and the decline in the use of antibiotics has led to interest in the use of immunosaccharides to reduce mortality and morbidity from digestive disorders. It is the author's belief that to date, this is the only published meta-analysis demonstrating the potential benefits of a feed additive (AGP included) on the growth performance and mortality of rabbits. The summary of the meta-analysis on the effects of Bio-Mos® in rabbit diets is presented in Table 4. Supplementing postweaning rabbit diets with an immunosaccharide (Bio-Mos®) significantly improved growth performance (weight gain and FCR) and liveability compared with a negative control. Diets supplemented with Bio-Mos® were statistically equivalent to diets containing AGP with regard to body weight gain and FCR. However in 9 comparisons Bio-Mos® tended to improve liveability to a greater extent (-28.7% reduction in mortality) compared with the AGP control diet. However, further studies will be necessary to obtain more conclusive data on the benefits of Bio-Mos® compared with an AGP control diet.

Conclusions

Research in the area of immunosaccharides has clearly shown that modulation of the immune response will lead not only to improved overall health but also to improved animal performance. Feed additives that can enhance the animal's ability to defend against potential antigens will ultimately lead to better health and growth performance. Immunosaccharides derived from the outer cell wall of yeast (Bio-Mos®) have been widely researched and their potential to improve growth performance and liveability has been demonstrated in meta-analyses of trials on pigs, broilers, turkeys and rabbits. Future research will add to existing knowledge and make existing meta-analysis more conclusive as well as expand to further animal groups which will help livestock producers to recognise the benefits of immunosaccharides such as Bio-Mos® on animal health and performance and this will ultimately reduce costs of livestock production.

References

Davis, M.E., Maxwell, C.V., Erf G.F., Brown, D.C. and Wistuba, T.J. (2004) Dietary supplementation with phosphorylated mannans improves growth response and modulates immune function of weanling pigs. *Journal of Animal Science* **82**: 1882–1891.

Ferket, P.R. (2004) Alternatives to antibiotics in poultry production: responses, practical experience and recommendations. In: *Biotechnology in the Feed Industry*. Edited by TP Lyons and KA Jacques. pp. 57-67. Nottingham University Press, Nottingham, UK.

Fioramonti, J., Theodorou, V. and Bueno, L. (2003) Probiotics: what are they? What are their effects on gut physiology? *Best Practice & Research Clinical Gastroenterology* **17**: 711-724.

Firon, N., Ofek, I. and Sharon, N. (1983) Carbohydrate specificity of the surface lectins of Escherichia coli, Klebsiella pneumoniae, and Salmonella typhimurium. *Carbohydrate Research* **120**: 235-249.

Hooge, D. (2004a) Meta-analyses of broiler chicken pen trials evaluating dietary mannan oligosaccharide, 1993-2003. *International Journal of Poultry Science* **3**: 163-174.

Hooge, D. (2004b) Turkey pen trials with dietary mannan oligosaccharide: meta-analysis, 1993-2003. *International Journal of Poultry Science* **3**: 179-188.

Hooge, D. and Sefton, A.E. (2004) Performance evaluation of dietary mannan oligosaccharide for broiler chickens: Ten years of field trials analyzed. In: *World Poultry Congress*. Istanbul, Turkey p. 529. (WPSA)

Klasing, K.C. (1998) Nutritional modulation of resistance to infectious diseases. *Poultry Science* **77**: 1119-1125.

Kocher, A., Spring, P. and Hooge, D. (2004) Rabbits may respond positively to dietary MOS. *Feedstuffs* **76**: 1-3.

Koutsos, E.A. and Klasing, K.C. (2001) Interactions between the Immune System, Nutrition, and Productivity of Animals. In: *Recent Advances in Animal Nutrition*. Edited by J Wiseman and PC Garnsworthy. pp. 173-190. Nottingham University Press, Nottingham

Koutsos, E.A. and Klasing, K.C. (2002) Modulation of nutritional status by the immune response. In: *Australian Poultry Science Symposium*. Sydney. Edited RAE Pym. pp. 18-23. University of Sydney

Moreau, M.C. and Gaboriau-Routhiau, V. (2000) Influence of resident intestinal microflora on the development and function's of the intestinal–associated lymphoid tissue. In: *Probiotics (3) Immunomodulation by the gut microflora and probiotics*. Edited by R Fuller and G Perdigon. pp. 69-114. Kluwer, London, UK.

Newman, K. (2004) Glycomics: putting carbohydrates to work for animal and human health. In: *Biotechnology in the Feed Industry*. Edited by TP Lyons and KA Jacques. pp. 27-32. Nottingham University Press.

Ofek, I., Mirelmann, D. and Sharon, N. (1977) Adherence of *Escherichia coli* to human cells mediated by mannose receptors. *Nature* **265**: 623-625.

O'Quinn, P.R., Funderburke, D.W. and Tibbetts, G.W. (2001) Effects of dietary supplementation with mannan oligosaccharides on sow and litter performance in commercial production systems. *Journal of Animal Science* **79**: 212.

Pettigrew, J.E. (2000) Mannan oligosaccharides' effects on performance reviewed. *Feedstuffs* **12**: 12-15.

Pettigrew, J.E. and Miguel, J.C. (2003) Meta-Analysis of the effect of Bio-Mos on nursery pig performance. *Feeding Times* **8**: 1-3.

Savage, G.P. and Zakrzewska, E.L. (1996) The performance of male turkeys fed a starter diet containing a mannan oligosaccharide (Bio-Mos) from day old to eight weeks of age. In: *Biotechnology in the Feed Industry*. Edited by TP Lyons and KA Jacques. pp. 47-54. Nottingham University Press, Nottingham, UK

Schmidt, K. (2002) Sugar rush. *New Scientist* **176**: 34.

Index

Lightning Source UK Ltd.
Milton Keynes UK
UKOW04f0732140517
301026UK00001B/20/P